About the author:

Jenny Morris is a disabled feminist and freelance writer/
researcher. She taught housing policy and sociology for
six years before giving up the struggle against disablism
within her workplace. She now puts her energies into
research and writing which gives a voice to disabled people.
This includes research consultancy work for local
authorities, working with Shelter on housing and disability
and doing a variety of other work around social policy
and disabled people.

She edited *Able Lives: Women's Experience of Paralysis*
(The Women's Press, 1989) and *Alone Together: Voices
of Single Mothers* (The Women's Press, 1992). She has
written a play entitled *Caring*.

About the book:

'A powerful polemic.' *The Observer*

'Recommended reading.' *Disability News*

'A refreshing, challenging read.' *Link*

'An important book . . . informative, uplifting and
empowering.' *The Northern Star*

Also by Jenny Morris from The Women's Press:

Able Lives: Women's Experience of Paralysis ed (1989)

Alone Together: Voices of Single Mothers ed (1992)

Also of interest:

Past Due: A Story of Disability, Pregnancy and Birth
Anne Finger (1991)

Pride Against Prejudice

A Personal Politics of Disability

Jenny Morris

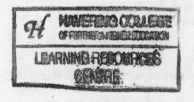

First published by The Women's Press Ltd, 1991
A member of the Namara Group
34 Great Sutton Street, London EC1V 0DX

Reprinted 1993

British Library Cataloguing-in-Publication Data
Morris, Jenny, *1950-*
  Pride against prejudice: transforming
  attitudes to disability
  I. Title
  362.4

ISBN 0 7043 4286 3

Phototypeset by Intype, London
Printed and bound in Great Britain by
BPCC Paperbacks Ltd
Member of BPCC Ltd

Contents

Acknowledgements

I am greatly indebted to the eight women who shared their thoughts about disability with me and whose words I have used in this book: Rachel Cartwright, Pam Evans, Mary Lawson, Anna Mathison, Molly McIntosh, Ruth Moore, Clare Robson, Sheila Willis.

I would like to acknowledge the help of a number of women who discussed this book with me, read draft chapters and/or gave me things which they had themselves written: Ruth Bashall, Nasa Begum, Jane Campbell, Merry Cross, Millie Hill, Rachel Hurst, Lois Keith, Linda Laurie, Ann Macfarlane, Jane Nation, Joanna Owen, Sian Vasey, Rosalie Wilkins.

I thank Jen Green for being so supportive and constructive in her editorial role and also thank her and Linda Laurie for the title.

Mandy Dee's poem is published by courtesy of her friend and literary executrix, Caroline Halliday, and Caroline's daughter, Kezia. The poem was first published in *Sinister Wisdom*, 39, (Winter 1989/90). Susan Hansell's poem is published by kind permission of Susan Hansell and has previously been published in *With the Power of Each Breath*, *Sinister Wisdom*, 32, (Summer 1987), and in *Kaleidoscope*, 10 (Spring 1985) and *Kaleidoscope*, 20 (Winter/Spring 1990).

To Pam Evans, in appreciation of her generosity;
and in loving memory of Liz Waugh

Introduction

Disabled people throughout the world are increasingly naming and confronting the prejudice which we daily experience, expressing our anger at the discrimination we face, and insisting that our lives have value. This book has grown out of the struggles through which, over the last decade or so, disabled people, and particularly disabled women, have asserted our reality. It is an attempt to analyse the nature of the prejudice we experience and to articulate the growing strength of our pride in ourselves.

It has also been within the last decade that I myself developed an identity as a disabled woman, an identity which has been a source of much anger at the prejudice and discrimination that I and other disabled people face. But it is also an identity which has been an increasing source of strength and liberation.

Beginnings

My own personal history as a disabled woman began in June 1983. I was feeling generally good about my life when, on a fine summer evening, I went out to mow the grass in the pocket handkerchief of my new garden that I was so proud of. My one year old daughter was asleep in her cot. Just before I switched on the lawnmower that I had borrowed from a friend I heard a child screaming. The sound came from the other side of the garden wall where there was a railway cutting. When I looked over the wall, I saw a small girl about three or four years old, standing on a ledge with a 20 foot drop below her to the railway line.

It didn't seem dangerous to step from the top of the wall on to the ledge to try to help her. But I fell and landed at the side of the railway track. (Someone else rescued the child.) At the moment of impact I lost all sensation in my legs.

Within the next few minutes I realised that I had broken my back. I don't know where the knowledge came from; I wasn't aware that I knew about spinal cord injury, paralysis and wheelchairs. But by the time the ambulance men arrived I had already worked out that I would not be able to convert my two bedroom council maisonette, of which I had been so pleased and proud, for using a wheelchair.

I didn't fully realise it then, but by stepping over that wall I became someone whose physical condition others feared. The acute physical pain that I experienced in the following days and the paralysis which it was soon clear would be permanent were too awful for many people to contemplate. They therefore used a variety of defence mechanisms to prevent themselves from having to identify with my reality. These defence mechanisms all took the form of people separating themselves off from me. Sometimes this was achieved by believing that I had somehow brought my paralysis on myself – as when the hospital nurses assumed that I had attempted suicide and thrown myself off the wall. Often it was a denial of the pain I was experiencing – it's very difficult to acknowledge another's physical pain, especially when there is nothing you can do about it.

I became aware that other people's refusal to take on my subjective reality was also linked to an assumption that was held by many I came in contact with. In subtle and not so subtle ways a number of people conveyed to me that they felt my life was no longer worth living. I remember feeling outraged that the doctor who sat down at my bedside with a gloomy face, to tell me that I was permanently paralysed, should talk about how 'tragic' it was. I felt that there was only one person who could say it was a tragedy and that was me – and I wasn't prepared to say that. He wittered on about incontinence and spasms but I didn't really take it in. I was so offended that he seemed to be writing off my life.

The consultant had a more practical attitude, which was closer to mine. Yes, I was paralysed, he said, but I would be 'very mobile, very mobile indeed'. I didn't understand the details of what he meant because I didn't at that point realise the enormous potential for physical independence that there is for a low-level paraplegic. But I understood the sense of what he was saying, and it fitted in with my perspective that losing the use of my legs was not by any means a tragedy.

The grief that I felt was more to do with my separation from my daughter and the break in my, at the point of my accident, highly satisfactory life. I had had a turbulent and often unhappy childhood, adolescence and early adulthood. But by the age of 33, things had consolidated into a fairly self-contained contentment. I had gone to university in my mid-twenties and then, after a few stops and starts, had completed a PhD. I had been a Labour councillor in Islington between 1978 and 1982, which had made me grow up quite a lot. I had finally got a flat of my own and found I loved living by myself. In May 1982 I had had a baby and the following month I had qualified as a teacher. My relationship with my daughter's father had ended fairly acrimoniously (because I had really wanted a child on my own), but he wanted to be a father and regularly looked after her. I had been living on Supplementary Benefit for the first year of Rosa's life because I enjoyed looking after her, but I had done a bit of part-time teaching at a further education college and had just accepted a full-time post which was to start in September, 1983. At that point Rosa would be 15 months old and, having organised a highly recommended childminder, I was feeling pleased with how things were working out.

It seemed so unfair that by stepping over that wall I had jeopardised all this. At the time, lying there in hospital, my terror was not about disability as such, but that I might have destroyed the structure of my life. However, this terror didn't last long. I resolved that the structure I had built would remain unchanged. All that had happened was that I would now be doing things from a sitting position. I just needed to sort things out in order to be able to do this. Little did I realise that by becoming paralysed I had become fundamentally different and set apart from the non-disabled world.

My friends were wonderful after my accident. Many of them started to take on the issues concerning disability at the same moment as I did – while I was still lying in bed at Stoke Mandeville hospital. I remember my friend Eileen recounting how she had challenged another Labour Party member who had been bewailing the tragedy of my accident, by arguing that most of my life was spent sitting down anyway (not least in Labour Party meetings) so being in a wheelchair wouldn't make much difference. And I remember Jane saying that if ever there was a time in history when it was exciting to be disabled it must be now, when disabled people were starting to organise, challenge the prejudice they experienced and demand their right to a decent quality of life.

At the time, such positive reactions to my new state seemed an inevitable part of my friends' socialism and feminism. It was only later – when I came to understand the depth and strength of prejudice and fear of disability – that I realised how unusual their affirming support for me was.

I had been active in the trades union and labour movement, and in the women's movement, all my adult life. When I became disabled I looked to these movements to help me make sense of my new experience. In particular I looked to feminism – with its central tenet of 'the personal is political' – to translate my subjective experience into a wider social and economic context.

Feminism

In 1971, when I was 21 years old, my identity, perceptions and assumptions about the world had been fundamentally challenged. The bewildering experience of my adolescence suddenly made sense and my feelings of isolation were replaced by a powerful sense of togetherness. In other words, I discovered feminism. The deep sense of unease which I had felt since puberty was suddenly articulated by the realisation that my awareness of being excluded, my sense of a rigid, powerful set of ideas imposing itself on me was not an isolated, individual experience but was rooted in what it means to be a woman in a male-dominated society.

During the 1970s the wealth of feminist expression – from Sheila Rowbotham's work to the plays of Monstrous Regiment – empowered me to gain an autonomy which I would never otherwise have known. I was both angry and joyful. Relationships with men became difficult and sometimes impossible, but a women-centred existence was wonderful. Feminism as a belief system decoded my social experience and my own attitudes. It gave me validity and legitimised the life I chose.

For women like me, as Liz Stanley and Sue Wise write, feminism is a way of living our lives.

> It occurs as and when women, individually and together, hesitantly and rampantly, joyously and with deep sorrow, come to see our lives differently and to reject externally imposed frames of reference for understanding these lives, instead beginning the slow process of constructing our own ways of seeing them, understanding them, and living them. For us, the insistence on the deeply political nature of everyday life and on seeing political change as personal change, is quite simply, 'feminism' (L Stanley and S Wise, 1983, p. 192).

One of the important results of the rise of feminism during the 1970s was its impact on the academic world. Feminist academics challenged the traditional ways in which research was done and experiences explained, and in so doing changed the way that both men and women saw themselves.

Feminist research has undergone two stages in its development over the last 20 years. The first was that of 'adding women in' to the previously male-dominated view of the world. This produced some revealing studies in a number of different disciplines, but it was the second stage which was more revolutionary. Feminists found that, rather than just adding women to the subject matter of research, theories and methodologies had to be fundamentally challenged, because existing models and paradigms were inadequate to explain women's (or men's) realities.

As Bari Watkins writes,

> Feminist scholars found that you could not simply add women to fields where they had previously been ignored. The models and paradigms of existing scholarship did not simply leave women out; they did not permit satisfactory explanations of women's experiences. They painted a picture of the world which was basically wrong or misguided because women's lives did not fit into its outlines. It was

therefore necessary to transform and reconstruct traditional ideas and methods in order to include women (Bari Watkins, 1983, pp. 81–82).

In so doing, feminists not only asserted that the personal, subjective experience of women was a legitimate area of research but that how this research was done had to be revolutionised. They went on to develop new paradigms, theories and, finally, a new philosophy which illustrated that feminism is not just about the study of women but about an entirely new way of looking at the world (see, for example, Diana Fuss (1989), Jean Grimshaw (1986), Caroline Ramazanoglu (1989), Elizabeth Spelman (1990).

The most recent developments in feminist thought have focused on a recognition of the experiences of different groups of women and the relationship between gender and other forms of oppression. Elizabeth Spelman, among others, has argued that feminism's assertion of what women have in common has almost always been a description of white middle-class women, and that when other groups of women are considered they tend to be 'added on' as subjects of research and theorising. White middle-class women's experiences have been taken as the norm and other women's experiences have been treated as 'different', as the subject of particular study and analysis. Thus, white middle-class women reality is the basis of general theory and analysis (in same way that men's reality was), and the reality of other groups of women is treated as particular, as separate from the general.

Spelman writes, for example,

Most philosophical accounts of 'man's nature' are not about women at all. But neither are most feminist accounts of 'woman's nature', or 'women's experiences' about all women. There are startling parallels between what feminists find disappointing and insulting in western philosophical thought and what many women have found troubling in much of western feminism (E Spelman, 1990, p. 6).

Such a recognition has (potentially) as radical an effect on feminist thought as feminism itself has had on world views dominated by men and men's experiences.

Serious omissions

Yet there are two groups of women who are missing from Spelman's analysis, as from feminist thought generally. In identifying that 'working class women, lesbian women, Jewish women and women of colour' have been considered as 'inessential' within feminist philosophy, Spelman has – in common with most non-disabled feminists – left out two important groups, namely older women and disabled women. Disability and old age are aspects of identity with which gender is very much entwined but they are identities which have been almost entirely ignored by feminists.

Feminist theory has been broadened, and refined, by the placing of the issues of class and race at the heart of feminism as a philosophy and as explanation. But the issues of disability and old age are either not considered at all, or dismissed in the way that Caroline Ramazanoglu does when she justifies her failure to incorporate disabled and older women into her analysis. She writes,

> while these are crucial areas of oppression for many women, they take different forms in different cultures, and so are difficult to generalise about. They are also forms of difference which could be transformed by changes in consciousness (C Ramazanoglu, 1989 p. 95).

These are really flimsy arguments. Racism also takes different forms in different cultures; yet recent feminist analysis has, quite rightly, argued that Black women's experiences and interests must be placed at the heart of feminist research and theory. Ramazangolu's second statement is an extraordinary denial of the socio-economic base of the oppression which older people and disabled people experience – we might as well say that racism can be eradicated by compulsory anti-racism training.

The fact that disability has not been integrated into feminist theory arises from one of the most significant problems with feminism's premise that 'the personal is political'. As Charlotte Bunch acknowledges,

> In looking at diversity among women, we see one of the weaknesses of the feminist concept: that the personal is political. It is valid that each woman begins from her personal experiences and it is important to see how these are political. But we must also recognise that our personal experiences are shaped by the culture with all its prejudices. We cannot therefore depend on our perception alone as the basis for political analysis and action – much less for coalition. Feminists must stretch beyond, challenging the limits of our own personal experiences by learning from the diversity of women's lives (C Bunch, 1988, p. 290).

Disabled people – men and women – have little opportunity to portray our own experiences within the general culture, or within radical political movements. Our experience is isolated, individualised; the definitions which society places on us centre on judgements of individual capacities and personalities. This lack of a voice, of the representation of our subjective reality, means that it is difficult for non-disabled feminists to incorporate our reality into their research and their theories, unless it is in terms of the way the non-disabled world sees us.

This does not mean that the experience of disability and old age should be 'added on' to existing feminist theory. Integrating these two aspects of identity into feminist thought will be just as revolutionary as feminism's political and theoretical challenge to the way that the experience of the white male was taken as representative of general human experience. Indeed feminism's challenge must remain incomplete while it excludes two such important aspects of human experience and modes of social and economic oppression.

This book is an attempt to further an understanding of the subjective reality of disability so that the diversity of women's experiences, which needs to be integrated into feminist research and theory, can also include our own.

Feminism and disability politics

This book is also an assertion that a feminist perspective has great relevance to disabled people generally and to disability politics. If ever 'the personal is political' was a fruitful and powerful concept it is in its application to the experience of disability. Susan Griffin has identified the way in which, during the 1970s, women

> asserted that our lives, as well as men's lives, were worthy of contemplation; that what we suffered in our lives was not always natural, but was instead the consequences of a political distribution of power. And finally, by these words, we said that the feelings we had of discomfort, dissatisfaction, grief, anger and rage were not madness, but sanity (S Griffin, 1982, p. 6).

The relevance of these words to disabled people shouts out to be recognised. Our anger is not about having 'a chip on your shoulder', our grief is not a 'failure to come to terms with disability'. Our dissatisfaction with our lives is not a personality defect but a sane response to the oppression which we experience.

I have not set out to write a book about 'women and disability'. Rather I have brought the perspective of feminism to an analysis of the experience of disability, using the principle of making the personal political as my primary analytical tool. Like other political movements, the disability movement, both in Britain and throughout the world, has tended to be dominated by men as both theoreticians and holders of important organisational posts. Both the movement and the development of a theory of disability have been the poorer for this as there has been an accompanying tendency to avoid confronting the personal experience of disability.

In recent years, the disability movement has argued against the medical model of disability which health and social services professionals (and the general public) tend to apply to us. Within this model, disabled people are reduced to the medical condition which accounts for their physical and/or intellectual characteristics and there is little or no account taken of the social and economic context in which people experience such medical conditions. Disability activists have therefore developed a social model of disability, arguing that it is environmental barriers and social attitudes which disable us. To put it very simply, it is not the inability to walk which disables someone but the steps into the building.

Such a perspective is a crucial part of our demand for our needs to be treated as a civil rights issue. However, there is a tendency within the social model of disability to deny the experience of our own bodies, insisting that our physical differences and restrictions are *entirely* socially created. While environmental barriers and social attitudes are a crucial part of our experience of disability – and do indeed disable us – to suggest that this is all there is to it is to deny the personal experience of physical or intellectual restrictions, of illness, of the fear of dying. A feminist perspective can help to redress this, and in so doing give voice to the experience of both disabled men and disabled women.

Writing this book

For me this book is both a personal exploration of the sources of my anger and a celebration of the strengths which have come from realising that I am now part of a movement which is making fundamental challenges to the kind of society in which we all live.

I have drawn extensively on the thoughts of other disabled people. These are not always to be found in the traditional cultural forms, for these are often closed to us. Disabled writers, film makers, playwrights, poets and others are developing our own culture, but it is non-disabled people's representations of disability which dominate the general culture.

As with other oppressed groups at the early stages of collective struggle, an oral tradition (or in the case of Deaf people, a signing tradition) is an important source of the passing on of ideas. This is partly why – at various points in the book – I have used the words of eight disabled women, who have been generous enough to share their thoughts with me, to help me to make sense of a number of different issues. I have used extracts from taped interviews with seven of the women, while one wrote down her thoughts on the various issues which I wanted to cover. I have interviewed women partly in order to redress the imbalance stemming from the fact that men's views and experiences are amply represented in the written material which also forms some of the resources for this book.

I have also used these women's words because my intention is to make our personal experience political, using an exploration of our subjective reality to assert the validity of our accounts as opposed to the way that non-disabled people view our lives. These eight women's experiences (although they cover a range of situations) are not intended to be representative of all disabled people, rather their words give expression to some of the issues which concern us.

The eight women (some of whom use pseudonyms) are:

Rachel Cartwright: Rachel was born blind. She is 74 years old. Her husband died five years ago. She has two children and three grandchildren and lives in Sheffield.

Pam Evans: Aged 45, Pam lives with her husband in a remote part of Shropshire. She has been a wheelchair user for over 20 years following a climbing accident when she was 18 years old.

Mary Lawson: Mary is 30 years old. She became completely paralysed in her early twenties as the result of an operation. She has spent some time in residential care and is now living in her own flat.

Anna Mathison: Anna was born disabled. She has no use of her upper limbs and uses a wheelchair. She is from Grenada and lives in London. She is in her thirties.

Molly McIntosh: Molly is in her sixties. She has scars on her face as a result of a fire when she was a child. Molly became deaf as the result of meningitis a few years ago. She lives in Leeds.

Ruth Moore: Ruth became disabled at the age of four. She uses a wheelchair and has limited use of her arms and hands. She is in her fifties.

Clare Robson: Clare has multiple sclerosis which was diagnosed seven years ago. She lives with her partner, Mo, who has two children.

Sheila Willis: Sheila has multiple sclerosis and lives with her daughter and her mother. She is 41 years old.

All these women have a physical or sensory disability. However, the issues discussed in this book also relate to learning disability. The non-disabled world is much concerned with *causes* of disability while the disability movement focuses on the effects and thus on our common experience of prejudice and discrimination. There are occasions when we need to pay particular attention to particular disabilities but this book is not one of them. In a similar fashion, Black disabled people and disabled gay men and lesbians express their particular concerns in particular contexts. This book attempts to integrate such concerns into its analysis: the experiences of such groups should not be treated as an 'added on' optional extra to a more general analysis of disability. Rather their experiences and interests are an integral part of the reality with which I am dealing.

Structure of the book

I begin by looking at our everyday experience of prejudice, examining our feelings about the way others behave towards us and at the same time trying to understand why they behave as they do. This is something that all of us grapple with and the thoughts of the eight women I have interviewed have been helpful in enabling me to understand the nature of prejudice.

The widespread assumption that disabled people's lives are not worth living, an important part of our experience of prejudice, is the subject of the second chapter. This chapter makes links between the contemporary experience of prejudice and the wholesale slaughter of disabled people in Hitler's Germany. Recent research has exposed the way that doctors in the Third Reich held that the quality of life for disabled people was, inevitably, so poor that to end such lives was 'mercy killing'. Such a judgement is also at the heart of the recent 'assisted suicide' cases in the USA and, using a variety of sources of material, I explore such attitudes in both Britain and the USA.

Arguments that the quality of disabled people's lives is so poor as to warrant 'mercy killing' have not been confined to adults but have also been applied to disabled children, babies, foetuses and to the prevention of disability. I therefore found that I also had to confront the potential conflict between disabled and non-disabled feminists on the issues of abortion and 'allowing' disabled babies to die. This is the subject of chapter 3. This was not an easy chapter to write but these are issues which women and disabled people must resolve and they throw up a number of wider questions.

Assumptions that our lives are not worth living are only possible when our subjective realities find no place in mainstream culture. Where disability is represented in the general culture it is primarily from the point of view of the non-disabled and so their fears and hostility, and their own cultural agendas, dominate the way we are presented. Chapter 4 addresses this, looking particularly at representations of disability in some recent films and plays and at the way that notions of masculinity and femininity are a crucial part of such representations. The chapter also looks at the way charities represent disabled people and at the attitude of advertisers to disability.

Chapter 5 looks at our experience of society's responses to some of the needs created by our physical and intellectual differences, showing how an unequal power relationship between disabled and non-disabled people creates both oppression and a denial of that oppression. I discuss both the experience of institutionalisation and research on 'residential care'. The chapter also discusses concepts of dependence and independence and addresses the question of what resources we need to live the kind of lives we choose.

The issue of resources is very much bound up with the political debates about 'community care', a subject to which feminists have made an important contribution by highlighting the lives of those who care for elderly and disabled relatives. Chapter 6 looks at this feminist research and analysis from the point of view of disabled people – one which has been entirely missing from the debate.

Finally, chapter 7 addresses the meaning of disability, the collective organisations of disabled people, the strengths we can draw from each other and the issues that we have to tackle if we are to further the interests of all disabled people.

This book was driven by the anger and hurt I experience as a result of prejudice and discrimination. But it was also motivated by a tremendous sense of powerfulness which has come from my contact with other disabled women, both in person and through their writings and other work. As women and as disabled people, we have an important contribution to make to feminist culture, to disability culture and also to the general culture. So I would hope that this book is also a celebration of our strength and a part of our taking pride in ourselves, a pride which incorporates our disability and values it.

Chapter 1:
Prejudice

This chapter is concerned with our experience of non-disabled people's reactions to physical and intellectual differences and how these reactions affect us, particularly in the way we feel about ourselves.

During the years following my accident, I have on countless occasions been told by both strangers and acquaintances how 'wonderful' they think I am. It took a while to realise why this kind of remark provoked such anger in me. After all, those who say it seem to think that they are praising me for struggling against the difficulties which physical disability brings. When I eventually unpeeled the layers of patronising nonsense I realised that at the heart of such remarks lay the judgement that being disabled must be awful, indeed intolerable. It is very undermining to recognise that people look at me and see an existence, an experience, which they would do everything to avoid for themselves.

How can we take pride in ourselves, in what we are, when disability provokes such negative feelings among non-disabled people? In order to start to answer this question disabled people have developed an understanding of the nature of prejudice and its effect on us.

Normality and difference

In our society, prejudice is associated with the recognition of difference and an integral part of this is the concept of normality. There are various ways of using the word normal. In theory it could be a value-free word to mean merely that which is common, and to be different from normal would not therefore necessarily provoke prejudice. In practice, of course, there are very strong values tied up with what our society considers to be normal and abnormal. Pam Evans, one of the women who shared her thoughts with me for this book, points out that the idea of normality is inherently tied up with ideas about what is right, what is desirable and what belongs.

She told me,

> Normal implies that which is average within any social structure. Those who do not conform to what is average in terms of appearance, function, behaviour or belief are no longer 'normal'. The degree to which they fail to conform indicates the scale on which they will be mistrusted, feared and finally rejected. They are 'other', 'alien'. They do not 'belong' because they no longer represent the collective values of the status quo. They challenge the way in which their society is certain it is right and admirable to be.
>
> There was a renowned Cambridge don who hated being obliged to respond to aimless chat on long air journeys. So, before embarking he would wind a piece of string around one ear and place the loose end in the side of his mouth. This simple device ensured that only the air hostess would dare address him. This may seem simply an amusing anecdote but what it tells us of human nature is infinitely instructive. The gulf between being regarded as normal or abnormal is as small as what you choose to make of a piece of string.

It is quite clear that – in the sense, that Pam Evans is using the word – disabled people are not normal in the eyes of non-disabled people. Our difference is measured against normality and found wanting. Our physical and intellectual characteristics are not 'right' nor 'admirable' and we do not 'belong'. It is particularly important to state this because – having given such a negative meaning to abnormality – the non-disabled world assumes that we wish to be normal, or to be treated as if we were. From this follows the view that it is progressive and liberating to ignore our differences because these differences have such negative meanings for non-disabled people. But we *are* different. We reject the meanings that the non-disabled world attaches to disability but we do not reject the differences which are such an important part of our identities.

We can assert the importance of our experience for the whole of society, and insist on our rights to be integrated within our communities. However, it is important that we are explicit about the ways in which we are not like the non-disabled world. By claiming our own definitions of disability we can take pride in our abnormality, our difference.

It is also important to understand the experience of being different in the context of the prejudice that is evoked by disability.

The experience of being different

There are two factors which need separating out when considering the relationship of disabled people to what is considered to be normal. First, we are often physically different from what is considered to be the norm, the average person. A feminist photographer once told me that her motivation for mounting an exhibition on lesbian mothers was 'to show that lesbians didn't have two heads!' The point is that disabled people *do*, or at least the social equivalent. Our bodies generally look and behave differently from most other people's (even if we have an invisible physical disability there is usually something about the way our bodies behave which gives our difference away). It is not normal to have difficulty walking or to be unable to walk; it is not normal to be unable to see, to hear; it is not normal to be incontinent, to have fits, to experience extreme tiredness, to be in constant pain; it is not normal to have a limb or limbs missing. If we have a learning disability the way we interact with others usually reveals our difference.

These are the types of intellectual and physical characteristics which distinguish our experience from that of the majority of the population. They are all part of the human experience but they are not the norm; that is, most people at any one point in time do not experience them, although many may experience them at some point in their lives.

The second part of our experience which distinguishes us from the norm is the way in which our physical and intellectual characteristics often mean that we have additional needs which have to be met if we are to have a reasonable quality of life. These needs may take a number of different forms: housing, heating, help with personal care, equipment, drugs and other medical treatment, technological or human help with communication, and so on.

We can assert our rights to the things that will enable us to have a good quality of life – the right to a home, to choose our personal relationships, to have children, to be economically independent. But it is important to recognise that our differences are significant both in terms of what we require to make these things possible and also in terms of the non-disabled world's reaction to these requirements.

I will be discussing later in this book some of the ways in which reactions to our differences can result in physical and emotional abuse and can indeed threaten our very lives. Prejudice lies at the heart of the segregation which many disabled people experience both as children and as adults. However prejudice can also take more subtle forms and in these cases is often more difficult to both name and fight against. As Pam Evans says, 'We have all experienced open hostility. On the whole it isn't very common, and is in any case easier to cope with, because it is out in the open and is readily seen by the able-bodied to be unacceptable and offensive behaviour.'

The manifestations of prejudice which can also have an important impact on our lives are often not out in the open; they are the hidden assumptions about us which form the bedrock to most of our interactions with the non-disabled world. It is often difficult for us to identify *why* someone's behaviour makes us so angry, or feel undermined. Our anger and insecurity can thus seem unreasonable not just to others but also, sometimes, to ourselves.

From her interaction with non-disabled people, Pam Evans has identified a number of assumptions which are held about disabled men and women. It is useful to state these explicitly because, in general, the non-disabled world will try to deny these attitudes. From our point of view, however, our experience of interacting with non-disabled people is characterised by such assumptions. The list, as she says, is incomplete, but these ideas make up the essence of the prejudice which we experience on a day-to-day basis. The assumptions about us are:

That we feel ugly, inadequate and ashamed of our disability.

That our lives are a burden to us, barely worth living.

That we crave to be 'normal' and 'whole'.

That we are aware of ourselves as disabled in the same way that they are about us and have the same attitude to it.

That nothing can be gained from the experience.

That we constantly suffer and that any suffering is nasty, unjust and to be feared and retreated from.

That whatever we choose to do or think, any work or pursuit we undertake, is done so as 'therapy' with the sole intention of taking our mind off our condition.

That we don't have, and never have had, any real or significant experiences in the way that non-disabled people do.

That we are naive and lead sheltered lives.

That we can't ever really accept our condition, and if we appear to be leading a full and contented life, or are simply cheerful, we are 'just putting a good face on it'.

That we need 'taking out of ourselves', with diversions and rewards that only the normal world can provide.

That we desire to emulate and achieve normal behaviour and appearance in all things.

That we go about the daily necessities or pursue an interest because it is a 'challenge' through which we can 'prove' ourselves capable.

That we feel envy and resentment of the able bodied.

That we feel our condition is an unjust punishment.

That any emotion or distress we show can only be due to our disability and not to the same things that hurt and upset them.

That our disability has affected us psychologically, making us bitter and neurotic.

That it's quite amazing if we laugh, are cheerful and pleasant or show pleasure in other people's happiness.

That we are ashamed of our inabilities, our 'abnormalities' and loathe our wheelchairs, crutches or other aids.

That we never 'give up hope' of a cure.

That the inability to walk, to see or to hear is infinitely more dreadful than any other physical aspects of disability.

That we believe our lives are a 'write off'.

That words like 'walk' and 'dance' will upset us – as if people who've endured what we have endured have fragile sensibilities.

That when we affirm that we cannot, or do not wish to do something, our judgement and preferences are overridden and contradicted as inferior to theirs.

That we are asexual or at best sexually inadequate.

That we cannot ovulate, menstruate, conceive or give birth, have orgasms, erections, ejaculations or impregnate.

That if we are not married or in a long-term relationship it is because no one wants us and not through our personal choice to remain single or live alone.

That if we do not have a child it must be the cause of abject sorrow to us and likewise never through choice.

That any able-bodied person who marries us must have done so for one of the following suspicious motives and never through love: desire to hide his/her own inadequacies in the disabled partner's obvious ones; an altruistic and saintly desire to sacrifice their lives to our care; neurosis of some sort, or plain old fashioned fortune-hunting.

That if we have a partner who is also disabled, we chose each other for no other reason, and not for any other qualities we might possess. When we choose 'our own kind' in this way the able-bodied world feels relieved, until of course we wish to have children; then we're seen as irresponsible.

That if our marriage or relationship fails, it is entirely due to our disability and the difficult person this inevitably makes us, and never from the usual things that make any relationship fail.

That we haven't got a right to an able-bodied partner, and that if they happen to be very obviously attractive, it's even more of a 'waste'.

That any able-bodied partner we have is doing us a favour and that we bring nothing to the relationship.

That we can't actually *do* anything. That we 'sit around' all day 'doing nothing'. Sitting seems to imply resting so it is presumed that we get no 'exercise'.

That those of us whose disability is such that we require a carer to attend to our physical needs are helpless cabbages who don't *do* anything either and have nothing to give and who lead meaningless, empty lives.

That if we are particularly gifted, successful or attractive before the onset of disability our fate is infinitely more 'tragic' than if we were none of these things.

That we should put up with any inconvenience, discomfort or indignity in order to participate in 'normal' activities and events. And this will somehow 'do us good'.

That our only true scale of merit and success is to judge ourselves by the standards of their world.

That our need and right to privacy isn't as important as theirs and that our lives need to be monitored in a way that deprives us of privacy and choice.

That we are sweet, deprived little souls who need to be compensated with treats, presents and praise.

As Ruth Bashall, a disabled lesbian who read a draft of this chapter, pointed out to me, we could add the assumption that disabled people could not possibly be lesbians or gay and that if we are this is because we cannot achieve a 'normal' heterosexual relationship rather than being an expression of our sexuality. Nasa Begum, a disabled Asian woman, drew my attention to some of the assumptions imposed on black and ethnic minority disabled people. These include the assumptions that, as she put it, 'it is our ethnic culture which restricts our lives as disabled people and that 'we should be grateful for the services we receive in Western societies, because we wouldn't be able to get them in our own countries.'

One of the biggest problems for disabled people is that all these undermining messages, which we receive every day of our lives from the non-disabled world which surrounds us, become part of our way of thinking about ourselves and/or our thinking about other disabled people. This internalisation of *their* values about *our* lives is discussed later.

Another important point to make is that, although Pam Evans is right in that overt hostility is not a common experience for most disabled people, it is yet the iron fist in the velvet glove of the patronising and seemingly benevolent attitudes which we experience. This is clear from the experience of those of us who step out of the passive role which society accords to us. In these situations we often have to confront dislike, revulsion and fear. When I interviewed Ruth Moore she talked about when she started running Disability Equality training a few years ago. Her experience of the hostility which some non-disabled people on her courses expressed towards disabled people was such a shock that she had to seek help in dealing with the emotional consequences for her.

The hostility was not directed towards me as an individual but towards disabled people. I never dreamed that there was such a subconscious, *and* conscious, degree of hatred

– the hatred expressed by the people I was training was far more powerful than their patronising attitudes. I was really surprised and shocked. I had come from such a traditional background of experiencing patronisation. And to come from that to realise that I was also a person who was hated. I was most fortunate to obtain some help. I had to rush around finding some professional help in order to survive.

The importance of physical difference

The prejudice that we experience is often a reaction to physical difference rather than a reaction to physical limitations. An obituary for David Rappaport, an actor who was three feet eleven inches tall and who committed suicide, made this point.

> Rappaport's death suggests quite powerfully that the continuing rejection of people with disabilities has little to do with physical limitations, often a justification of their shabby treatment. His death suggests that being physically different is the key to a whole range of biases in our increasingly physicalist society (Bill Bolte, 1990).

Bolte believes that the situation (in America at least) has worsened in recent years.

> Though I choose to live now at wheelchair height, I understand why David Rappaport chose death. He could no longer carry the burden of being different (and considered defective) in a world that increasingly worships a standardised sense of physical acceptability. He could no longer carry the additional burden of trying to pass.

When I talked to Molly McIntosh, who has no physical limitations but who has a clear physical difference, she explained how her life has been almost completely determined by other people's reactions to this physical difference.

I have horrible scars on my face. What I mean by that is

that people react to them with horror. Forty years ago, when I was in my twenties, and also when I was a child, I *so* hated the way that I looked. I tried not to think about it but every time I went out in the street I would be reminded about how I looked because of the way people reacted to me. As I walked down the street and someone was coming towards me, they would look and then drop their eyes or move their head, as if the horror was too much. But then they could never, ever resist looking again. I used to have bets with myself about that second look. I would promise myself a treat if they didn't look again but they always did.

Molly was badly burned when a child. She also has scars on the upper part of her body but the prejudice she experiences is through people's reactions to her face.

I felt very lonely as a child. I never remember having children from school home to play – or going to their houses. My brothers and sister did but not me. Whenever I got bullied in the playground it was always in terms of insults about my face. I felt the teachers didn't want to deal with that; they never did anything about the way other children reacted towards me and anyway they themselves found it difficult to look me in the eye. When I left school, I did a typing course but found it difficult to get work. Typists were supposed to be attractive and cheerful and I was ugly and miserable. Even when I could get work, I just hated the way people reacted towards me when they first met me. In the end, my mother said I may as well stay at home and help her with the housework because she had got herself a part-time job. I started to enjoy my life more then. I got very good at cooking and started to help my father in the garden. By the time he died I was more or less running the household and then when Mum became ill I took over everything.

Molly McIntosh felt that her life was split in two. When she was at home she felt at ease with herself. She limited her excursions into the outside world to the local shops, the library and the garden centre.

> People who I saw once a week or so, in the local shops and things, tried to pretend that they had no reaction to my face, Maybe they *did* become so used to me they didn't think about it. I don't think so though. They were friendly enough but I never felt treated as an equal. I was 'that poor woman down the road, you know, the one with the *FACE*' (the last phrase spoken in a whisper). Of course, I never heard them say that, but you *feel* the way that other people think about you. And I never felt other than different.

Every time therefore that Molly set foot outside her front door, she felt a sense of unease.

Most of us experience this same sense of unease each time we interact with the non-disabled world, particularly in a public situation where we are dealing with strangers' reactions to us. Tina Leslie, who like Molly McIntosh has scars on her face, gave voice to this feeling and the profound effect it can have on our sense of self, in the film *The Fifth Gospel* screened by BBC's Everyman series:

> At home with my family, with my animals, with my lover, I don't feel they condemn me for this mask. And so for a short while I'm allowed to be me, the real me . . . I only cease to be the person I know I am when I walk down the street. Then I see the look in your eyes. I see your horror and your revulsion. It's like being cut in half.

Going out in public so often takes courage. How many of us find that we can't dredge up the strength to do it day after day, week after week, year after year, a lifetime of rejection and revulsion? It is not only physical limitations that restrict us to our homes and those whom we know. It is the knowledge that each entry into the public world will be dominated by stares, by condescension, by pity and by hostility.

Some of us find that the only way we can survive in a non-disabled world is either not to recognise how much we are feared and hated, or to pretend that we don't know about it.

As one American disabled woman wrote,

> I pretend to forget how deeply disabled people are hated. I pretend to forget how this is true even within my chosen home, the lesbian and feminist communities. My survival at every level depends on maintaining good relationships with able-bodied people (Sandra Lambert, 1989 p.72).

Some of us feel that we can confront the stares and hostility head on. I talked to Anna Mathison who lives within a Black community in which she feels she belongs. She has the confidence to refuse to be intimidated by other people's reactions to her as someone with a very visible disability. 'If people stare, I shout "What are you staring at? You want to feel? You need glasses?" I feel I should challenge them because otherwise they think you're stupid and that they are entitled to stare.'

An experience that Anna had when she was 18 made a big impression on her attitude towards non-disabled people's reactions to physical difference. 'I was going down the Cheltenham Promenade with a girl I was at school with. She had a tumour on her face which made her look a bit like the "Elephant Man". These two women were coming towards us and they started staring. And as they passed us, one said "If I had a daughter like that, I wouldn't let her live." What do you do to women like that? You don't let them do it to you again. You don't let them get at you.'

However, Anna Mathison remains all too aware that people look at her and think her life is not worth living. 'They just see the wheelchair and they think, you'd be better off dead. And that's a problem because it hurts. But if I shout at them it makes me strong.'

We receive so many messages from the non-disabled world that we are not wanted, that we are considered less than human. For those with restricted mobility or sensory disabilities, the very physical environment tells us we don't belong. It tells us that we aren't wanted in the places that non-disabled people spend their lives – their homes, their schools and colleges, their workplaces, their leisure venues. The refusal to give Sign the status of a language means that Deaf people are forced to use a language suited to people with different biological characteristics. The refusal to give Braille the same status as printed material shuts out people with a visual impairment. As Susan Hannaford writes, 'For no access read Apartheid' (S Hannaford, 1985 p. 121).

Rachel Cartwright, who was born blind, talked to me about her experiences of exclusion.

> All through my childhood, I felt set apart from my brothers and sisters. I went to a different school and because it was a residential school I felt as if I wasn't part of my family a lot of the time. When my parents talked about our future, they always thought in different terms when it came to me. As a child and as an adult I've been very aware of being excluded by the way that most printed material is not available on tape or in Braille, and that if it is, it's only because a special effort has been made – for which I'm supposed to feel grateful.

Some of the practical consequences of the failure of the non-disabled world to allow us into their environment are examined in chapter five, but it is important to emphasise here that such exclusion gives us a clear message about the attitude of non-disabled people towards us.

This exclusion is associated with the way that our physical or intellectual differences make us less than human in the eyes of non-disabled people; we can be excluded from normal human activity because we are not normally human. A physically different body, or a body which behaves in a different way, means an incomplete body and this means that our very selves are similarly incomplete. This attitude is revealed by things such as an advertisement for artificial limbs which reads, 'For children born with missing limbs, myoelectric replacements offer a chance to lead *lives that are whole*.' (JoAnne Rome, 1989, p.37, emphasis in original). Non-disabled people's judgements about disability undermine our very existence for, as the next chapter explores in some detail, our lives are very often considered to be not worth living.

The messages we receive are very strong and clear and we have little access to different values which may place a more positive value on our bodies, our selves and our lives. Our self image is thus dominated by the non-disabled world's reactions to us. How can we feel good about our bodies and our selves when we have the kind of experiences that JoAnne Rome, who was born without a left hand or arm below the elbow, writes about.

> The word 'deformed' pounded in my brain, though in truth I thought my hook far uglier than my arm. I hated the shiny metal hook that in later years replaced the child's rubber one. Hated how it stood out, hated it and hid behind it, for it had become my armour and I felt vulnerable without it. This thing that was supposed to make me more acceptable, help me function just like everyone else. My 'helper'. I hid in that device and hated it, but I was unable to conceive of not wearing it. I felt it would be far worse for people to look in horror at my real arm as they did at the hook.

It wasn't just a question of people staring but also of the way that her missing arm determined the way people behaved towards her.

> I used to believe I owed an explanation to whomever demanded one. I felt fearful, intimidated, ashamed, out of control and outraged, yet 'what happened to your arm?' was not a question that I could choose to answer or not. I was a freak, an outsider, an 'other' and the world made it very clear that I owed them an explanation. I was also a little girl who was chased home from school with taunts of 'Captain Hook!' ringing in my ears, the object of whispers, stares and laughter . . . The domination and submission in the abled/disabled relationship was/is very powerful. This harassment is a fact of my life. I've heard 'mind if I ask you a stupid/personal question?' from sensitive lesbian psychotherapists, suburban housewives, boys

in gas stations, sales clerks, doctors, joggers, dykes in bars
and so on, ad infinitum. I detest it, it hurts, I feel like an
object of curiosity, not a woman with a head and a heart
and feelings that should matter (Rome, 1989 p.37).

Non-disabled people feel that our differentness gives them
the right to invade our privacy and make judgements about
our lives. Our physical characteristics evoke such strong feelings that people often have to express them in some way.
At the same time they feel able to impose their feelings on
us because we are not considered to be autonomous human
beings. One woman, contributing to the American book *No
More Stares*, described an incident which illustrates this –
the only unusual thing being that, for once, she was able to
think of a powerful retort.

I was riding the subway one day and this woman came up
to me, sat down by me and said, 'Oh, my God, it's such
a shame! Such a pretty girl, such ugly hands!' (My hands
and feet were deformed at birth; the condition is called
syndactylism.) So I said to her, 'So would it be better if I
were *all* ugly?' She giggled and mumbled something about
a tragedy. I said, 'I don't think it's such a tragedy. You
think my hands are ugly, you should see my feet!' and got
off at my stop (DREDF, 1982, p.14).

We often experience the fascination that non-disabled
people have with 'just how do you *manage*?' They have a
consuming curiosity about how we pee, how we shit, how
we have sex (*do* we have sex?) Many of us have experienced
the total stranger or slight acquaintance coming up and
asking us the most intimate things about our lives. Our physical difference makes our bodies public property. Clare
Robson experienced this when as – a result of having multiple
sclerosis – one side of her body started shaking and she had
to use a stick to help her to walk. 'People would come up
to me in the street and ask me what was wrong. If I told
them, they would say "Oh, how awful, there's no cure for
that, is there?" It's pity that motivates that kind of reaction,
not empathy. And also it's voyeurism.'

Looking at someone with a physical disability does not always feel so undermining to the disabled person. There is a difference between staring and gazing. As another young woman – quoted in *No More Stares* puts it,

> There are people who make me feel like I'm looking at myself in a mirror at the fun house. Like the people on the bus today – the starers.
>
> Now some people can look at me forever and I wouldn't care. Those are the people who seem to see, not just the best of me, but the *most* of me. They're not *staring*, they're *gazing*.
>
> A stare is kind of like a vampire bite – it sucks life out of you. A gaze is just the opposite – a love transfusion (DREDF, 1982, p. 50).

My own experience bears this out. I can rest my eyes on another disabled person whom I come across when I'm shopping. We can smile at each other, exchange a few words and feel good about our feeling of identifying with each other. Sometimes, of course, other disabled people avoid catching my eye because of the negative way that we are made to feel about ourselves out in public. It took me a long time after my accident to feel good about being out in public with other disabled people. For me the breakthrough came when I was leaving a meeting in the company of a disabled man. As we came towards the doors leading out of the building a woman rushed up, saying, 'Let me open the doors for you' (her attitude of '*Poor* things' written all over her face and oozing out of her voice). But, before she could push her way in front of us – as people trying to open doors do so often – the doors opened automatically. '*Oh!*' she cried, '*Isn't* that clever. How does it work?' 'I don't know,' I said, 'I'm not an electrician.' And we sailed through the doors, leaving her open-mouthed and superfluous.

Thinking about this incident afterwards I realised I felt a feeling of power which came from two sources – the feeling of solidarity with another disabled person at whom her pity was also directed, and the fact that, for once, the physical environment had been altered to suit people like me. The automatic doors meant that I did not have to accept help from someone whose help was offered on her terms and not mine.

Help and anger

When we interact with the non-disabled world it isn't just staring and people's feelings about our physical differences that we have to deal with. We also have to deal with the issue of help – the help which non-disabled people often offer us, and the help which some of us need in going about our daily lives.

Susan Hannaford takes the example of people rushing to open doors for someone in a wheelchair. She says that, just as men assume that they know what women want, so non-disabled people assume that they know what we want. It is this assumption that characterises the way in which people open doors for us. She asks non-disabled women,

> . . . who hasn't had a smiling man open a door? His expectations are that you want him to, that you want his help. Who hasn't been told that women are like this – women like men being nice to them, women like being told that they look nice, women don't like getting dirty, taking leading roles or being without a boyfriend . . . Do you, like men do about us, make assumptions about me? Do you assume I need help, like men assume we do?
>
> When I go out to places, the handicapist society's attitudes surround me, like a sexist one used to when I was a young girl – and still does. People rush to open doors and stand there smiling at me. I now either ignore them completely or stop and wait – after a few minutes it sinks in that I'm not going to go through the open door and they embarrassedly let it go, no doubt thinking I am a bitter and twisted case. How often have you felt like ignoring the opened door, the ladies first, the take my seat attitude? How often have you felt angry? (Hannaford, p.120.)

Hannaford is responding to what she identifies as 'condescension masked as help'. We face an additional problem in that some of us, sometimes, need someone to open the door for us, and provide us with other physical help, and we can therefore feel guilty about declining help because it may mean that another disabled person will not be offered help when they need it. By refusing help we are often labelled as having a 'chip on the shoulder' and a non-disabled person feels resentful and says to themselves, 'Well, that's the last time I offer help to a disabled person.' Our sense of responsibility to other disabled people who may suffer because of our anger makes it difficult to know what to do.

The problem is that the terms on which help is offered are often demeaning and oppressive. We can never take the giving of help for granted. Mary Lawson spoke to me about her experience of living in residential care. She felt that she had to be nice to the people who were helping her with the most intimate tasks otherwise they would refuse to do them, or do them in such a way which caused her pain or humiliation. 'I want them to want to help me so I've got somehow to make them like me . . . I felt if people didn't like me they would do things for me in a slapdash, cackhanded way.' Sometimes she forgot to be nice enough. For example, one night she was being lifted into bed by two care assistants when she noticed her shoes were still on. When she said 'Could you take my shoes off?' the care assistant responded by telling her to say please. As Mary said, 'I don't know whether the humiliation and anger I felt at saying "please" was worth the benefit of having my shoes taken off.'

Other people decide for us what kind of help we need and when we tell them that their help is either not needed or is inappropriate they can react with anger and hostility. The book *No More Stares* includes a story about a girl who walks with a brace.

It started when I fell down on the way to the bus this morning. I mean I'm used to falling down and I hardly ever hurt myself. I must relax or something like they say to do when you fall off a horse. But anyhow, I would have been OK except this couple came up to help me and when they saw the brace they went into this emergency medic routine and told me to 'lay flat'. I was so embarrassed. I tried to tell them I was all right and that I had a bus to catch. I was struggling to get up and they kept pushing me back so they could 'test for fractures' and while we were tussling, the bus drove by.

Then I lost it. I screamed at them to leave me alone. Well you would have thought I spat at them. It stopped them cold. Then *they* started to scream. 'Who do you think you are? We were only trying to help.' I thought they might call the cops but they walked away mumbling at me. I got my stuff together and had to stand at the bus stop (of course there's no bench) for 15 minutes waiting for the next bus and feeling horrible for getting mad at them. My parents have always told me to be polite when people ask me questions in the street. People don't mean to be stupid, etc. (DREDF, 1982, p. 12).

We have to be very tolerant of non-disabled people's behaviour towards us, either because we need their help or because we can't afford to provoke their hostility and anger. When we do, we feel guilty.

There is a fine line between the 'pity mixed with distaste' with which most people approach us and outright hostility – as we discover when we step out of the role of 'poor little cripple'. I was getting into my car one day, having done my weekly food shopping, when I was aware – as I am so often aware – that someone was standing staring at me. I was feeling stroppy and bad tempered that day so I didn't feel like ignoring him. Instead, I turned round and stared back. But this didn't bother him at all; he continued staring. So finally I said, what are you staring at? 'Oh, I was just wondering whether you needed any help,' he said. I retorted, 'Well it's not very helpful to stand there staring at me.' At which he exploded. I couldn't write here the expletives he used as they are too offensive. When his wife came up – he had been waiting for her outside the shop – she looked shocked at his language as he obviously didn't normally behave like that. But then, it's not normal for one of us to talk back.

It is often difficult for us to understand why we feel angry when people offer us help – even when we sometimes need help with a physical task. Our anger then becomes undermining because we feel unreasonable. We can start to believe the 'bitter and twisted' stereotype so often applied to us. Pam Evans calls anger 'the ungracious response to offers of apparent help', arguing that

> The reason for this response is likely to spring from the instinct that knows that the help on offer isn't quite what it seems: that it demands a return. This kind of 'help' is a way for those offering it to make themselves feel 'good'. Because they don't recognise their own motives, they project their demand for gratitude and the fact that we are being *used* to this end. We are obliged to participate in the charade by smiling our thanks and pretending that we are not being used. To do otherwise would be indefensible! We are then left with an infuriating sense of guilt at feeling so insulted by what to all outer appearances is an act of care and kindness. We have to indulge their illusion that they are giving, when in fact they are only taking.

Generally, people offer help because this makes them feel good about themselves. It isn't surprising therefore that if we refuse to fall in with this, to make them the gift of our gratitude, that they respond with shock, surprise and sometimes hostility. As Pam Evans says,

> When we respond in anger we are like the child in the story who knows that the King hasn't got any clothes on; our instinct tells us what is true. If we are wise, however, we don't throw that truth back in the face of the one offering help, for they are unaware of what they are doing and we are in no position to give them the insight. For a start, they don't want it, or anything else that is uncomfortable to question.

Wanting to be normal?

One of the most oppressive features of the prejudice which disabled people experience is the assumption that we want to be other than we are; that is, we want to be normal. Yet,

as Pam Evans says, 'Do we only have value, even to ourselves, in direct relation to how closely we can imitate
"normal" appearance, function, belief and behaviour?' The
only way in which it seems we can gain acceptance is to
emulate normality. Indeed, some non-disabled people, who
seek to promote the rights of disabled people, insist that
'they are just like you and me'. We may have the same
aspirations as non-disabled people (in terms of how we live
our lives) but quite patently we are not just like them in that
we have differences which distinguish us from the majority
of the population. Nevertheless the pressures on us to aspire
to be 'normal' are huge – 'friends and family all conspire
from the kindest and highest of intentions to ensure we make
the wrong choice,' says Pam. 'Better to betray ourselves than
them!'

One of the biggest obstacles to disabled people coming
together to demand an end to the discrimination we face, is
the way in which we feel pressure to take on the non-disabled
world's judgements about ourselves. This can make it very
difficult for us to associate with other disabled people.

This is illustrated by Anne Finger, an American feminist
who had polio when she was a child, writing about her first
attendance at a conference of post-polio people.

I sat for the first time in my life in a room filled with other
disabled people. I remember how nervous I felt. Mark
was sitting next to me, and I felt glad to have a blond-
haired, able-bodied lover at my side. I'd always gone to
'regular' schools; I'd been mainstreamed before there was
a word for it. I had moved through the world as a normal
person with a limp, and no thank you, I didn't need any
help, I could manage just fine. And, no, I was nothing
like 'them'. I wasn't whiny, or needy or self-pitying.

She describes the complexity of her emotions as she discovered a sense of solidarity with other disabled people but
at the same time felt a sense of horror that her level of
physical disability might become as high as some of the others
at the conference, which was on the complications of growing
older for people who have had polio.

I felt such commonality with the other people there who'd had polio. It was as if I had been living all my life in a foreign land, speaking a language that was not my native tongue. Here I was at last among people who understood, who understood without elaboration, explanation . . . I wanted to be able to embrace this community. And I wanted to be able to walk away from it, too. I wanted to be able to return to the world where I more or less passed for normal. Normal. Pass. Loaded words (Finger, 1990, pp. 16–17).

They are loaded words indeed. Just as Anne Finger used her non-disabled lover to try to pass herself as 'normal', so do many of us use our lovers, our children, our jobs to insist that really we are just like non-disabled people. I myself prefer to go shopping with my child because her presence at my side gives me, I mistakenly think, a passport into the world of normal people. To assert that I am a mother is to distance myself from the abnormality of being disabled. Some of us take pride in 'looking normal except for sitting down'. Very few of us feel able to celebrate our physical difference, although more of us do as the disability movement grows stronger.

Cynthia Rich describes the way that older people experience a similar pressure to 'pass'.

Passing – except as a consciously political tactic for carefully limited purposes – is one of the most serious threats to selfhood. We attempt, of course, to avoid the oppressor's hateful distortion of our identity and the real menace to our survival of his hatred. But meanwhile, our true identity, never acted out, can lose its substance, its meaning, even for ourselves. Denial to the outside world and relief at its success ('Very few people think of me as old as I am. They don't. People can't tell how old I am') blurs into denial of self (I'm always surprised when I look down and see all that gray hair, because I don't feel gray-headed) (B MacDonald and C Rich, 1983, p. 55).

As Rich points out, one way of passing – of denying what

we really are to the outside world – is to present ourselves as an exception to the category to which we otherwise belong. I may be disabled but I lead a normal life in that I live in my own house, earn my living, bring up my child, go out to dinner, to the theatre. How many times has a disabled person thought or said as a matter of pride, 'Well, of course, most of my friends are able bodied'? I can insist that I am not like other disabled people who attend day centres, go to special schools, live in residential care, are taken on holiday in groups. But this divides me from the oppressed group of which I am inevitably a member. The non-disabled world either reacts to me with prejudice and discrimination, or, by seemingly benevolently treating me as an exception, makes invisible my oppression. As Rich says, 'That division can compound my isolation as well as rendering me politically impotent' (p. 56). Being exceptional may defend an individual against the commonality of our oppression but it is dangerous in that it denies our very identity.

One of the most important features of our experience of prejudice is that we generally experience it as isolated individuals. Many of us spend most of our lives in the company of non-disabled people, whether in our families, with friends, in the workplace, at school, and so on. Most of the people we have dealings with, including our most intimate relationships, are not like us. It is therefore very difficult for us to recognise and challenge the values and judgements that are applied to us and our lives. Our ideas about disability and about ourselves are generally formed by those who are not disabled.

In this situation, the emergence of a disability culture is difficult but tremendously liberating. Such a culture enables us to recognise the pressure to pretend to be normal for the oppressive and impossible-to-achieve hurdle which it is. Most importantly, this culture challenges our own prejudices about ourselves, as well as those of the non-disabled culture. This is vital for, as Pam Evans says,

Just as no feminist would think of trying to change discriminatory laws and conventions of society without *first* changing her own attitudes to her personal inheritance of conditioning, so no disabled person should see liberation from prejudice as solely a matter of changing others. The *real* liberation is essentially our own. For we are all accomplices to the prejudice in exact proportion to the values and norms of our society that we are prepared to endorse.

We are *not* normal in the stunted terms the world chooses to define. But we are not obliged to adopt those definitions as standards to which we must aspire, or indeed, as something worth having in the first place.

Physical disability and illness are an important part of human experience. The non-disabled world may wish to try to ignore this and to react to physical difference by treating us as if we are not quite human, but we assert that our difference is both an essential part of human experience, and given the chance, can create important and different ways of looking at things.

One of the most undermining things about non-disabled people's assumptions about us is that they often assume that our lives are inevitably of a poor quality because of our disability. Sheila Willis talked to me about this:

I feel that most of the people I know think that my life has got immeasurably worse since I had the diagnosis of multiple sclerosis. In fact, it's got better. I'm not denying the difficulties but being told that I had this illness made me rethink what I was doing. I was able to get out of a very repressive relationship and to live just with Pat [her mother] and Lauren [her daughter] – which is wonderful, it's what I've always wanted. And not having to go to work every day is also wonderful, it's so liberating. The writing that I'm doing now, I would never have done if I hadn't been told that I had MS. And yet, if I told my able-bodied friends that I think my life has improved they would think I was mad, which makes me feel sad.

The assumptions that non-disabled people hold about the quality of our lives can pose enormous problems for us and this is explored in the next chapter.

Chapter 2:
'Lives not Worth Living'

In May 1990, a 31-year-old man, Kenneth Bergstedt, petitioned the Las Vegas courts for permission to 'end his painful existence'. The press reported that he was 'a 31-year-old quadriplegic hooked to a respirator for more than 20 years' for whom 'life was no longer worth living'. A psychiatrist backed up his application by telling the court that 'The quality of life for this man is very poor, moderated only by momentary distraction, but forever profaned by a future which offers no relief' (Mary Johnson, 1990, p. 16).

This case is but one of an increasing number which have occurred in the USA over the last few years. The first one to be taken up by the disability movement was that of Elizabeth Bouvia, who had cerebral palsy. Dr Paul Longmore, a historian who is also disabled wrote:

A 26-year-old woman, attractive and educated, checks herself into a hospital psychiatric unit announcing her wish to commit suicide. She reports that she has undergone two years of devastating emotional crises: the death of a brother, serious financial distress, withdrawal from graduate school because of discrimination, pregnancy and miscarriage and, most recently, the breakup of her marriage.

She also has a serious physical disability, which she says is the reason she wants to die.

Three psychiatric professionals ignore the series of emotional blows, concluding that she is mentally competent and that her decision for death is reasonable. They base their judgement on one fact alone – her physical handicap' (P Longmore, 1987, p. 195).

The judge who heard the Bouvia case pronounced ' . . . she must lie immobile, unable to exist except through the physical acts of others' and expressed the hope that her case would 'cause our society to deal realistically with the plight of those unfortunate individuals to whom death beckons as a welcome respite from suffering' (Longmore, 1987, p. 195).

A key question for the American courts in these cases has been whether the person petitioning for 'assisted suicide' is taking a rational decision, that is, whether their wish to die is determined by emotion or impulse, or whether it is a reasonable judgement based on a realistic assessment of their situation.

As disability activists like Paul Longmore and Mary Johnson have pointed out, this assessment is made by people who often have no experience of disability, are certainly not disabled themselves and who find it inconceivable that someone who is completely (or almost completely) paralysed and who may have to use a respirator even to breathe, can experience a life which is worth living.

It seems to be relatively easy for the non-disabled world to judge that people who require physical assistance to such a high degree are making a rational decision when they say they want to die. It has been left up to other disabled people to examine the social and economic context in which such decisions are made. The case of Larry McAfee, whose case hit the American press in 1989, illustrates the way in which it is not the physical disability itself but the social and economic circumstances of the experience which can lead to a diminished quality of life (*Disability Rag*, July/August 1990, pp. 11–12).

McAfee was aged 34 when a motorcycle accident resulted in complete paralysis and the need to use a ventilator. His insurance benefit (of $1 million) enabled him to employ personal care attendants in his own home for a period after his accident but when this ran out he was forced to enter a nursing home. He decided life wasn't worth living and tried turning his respirator off but couldn't cope with the feeling of suffocation. So he petitioned the courts to be allowed to be sedated while someone else unplugged his breathing apparatus.

In the event, he acquired a delay mechanism which would allow him to turn off the respirator himself and still allow for sedation, and the court ruled that he could not be stopped from doing so. Throughout the case and the publicity accorded to him, the general assumption was that McAfee's decision was a rational one based solely on the extent of his physical disability.

Yet when, as a result of the publicity, McAfee received an outpouring of support from disability activists, he decided to delay the decision to take his own life. What he really wanted was to live in his own home and to get a job. A disability organisation arranged for him to receive training in voice-activated computers and he received tentative offers of employment. However, at this point, his Medicare benefits (the more generous part of the American health benefit system) ran out and the less-generous Medicaid would not pay for his place at the nursing home which was equipped for people who use a respirator. The Georgia Medicaid regulations did not allow Medicaid benefits to be used on home care but McAfee, together with disability activists and organisations, tried to get a waiver to the regulations to allow him to hire care attendants in his own home.

The type of nursing home which was equipped for McAfee's needs cost between $475 to $650 per day (a level which could be paid by Medicare but not Medicaid). McAfee calculated it would cost $265 per day to pay for attendant services in his own home but Medicaid paid only $100 per day for residential care. The Georgia Department of Medical Assistance therefore rejected his proposal. McAfee was then admitted, temporarily and on a voluntary basis, to a psychiatric hospital. Anyone in his situation must be extremely depressed and upset.

The social and economic context of Kenneth Bergstedt's desire to die is also clear. His case was brought into the limelight when his 65-year-old father presented the Las Vegas court with an affidavit from his son that he 'had no encouraging expectations to look forward to from life, receives no enjoyment from life, lives with constant fears and apprehensions and is tired of suffering' (Johnson, 1990, pp. 18–19). But were these feelings about his life a result of his physical disability or a result of the situation in which he lived? Bergstedt was being looked after by his father who was disabled himself (he had lost a leg in an industrial accident), had high blood pressure and was scared of getting cancer or having a heart attack. Bergstedt was said to be worried that if anything happened to his father he would either die if left on his own in an emergency or be forced into residential care. The court ruled that Bergstedt's wish to die was rational given the level of his physical disability, with no consideration as to whether, if the context in which he experienced his physical disability were changed, his attitude to dying might have been very different.

The question is, in such a context, is the wish to die a so-called rational response to physical disability? Or is it a desperate response to isolated oppression? As Ed Roberts, head of the World Institute on Disability, said, 'It's not the respirator. It's money.' He explained, 'I've been on a respirator for 26 years and I watch these people's cases – they're just as dependent on a respirator as I am; the major difference is they know they're going to be forced to live in a nursing home – or they're already there – and I'm leading a quality life' (*Disability Rag*, September/October 1990, p. 21).

In America, the debate is couched in terms of civil rights. Elizabeth Bouvia received the help of the American Civil Liberties Union lawyers who were intent on winning for her the legal right to assisted suicide (Longmore, 1987, p. 195). It is also couched in terms of humanitarianism, of concern for the individual and their quality of life.

In Britain, where such cases rarely reach the courts, public opinion has also been concerned with the issue of quality of life for physically disabled people. There has been a similar willingness to accept that a high level of paralysis necessitates an unacceptable quality of life. One example of this involved James Haig, who was tetraplegic as the result of a motorbike accident. During the year following his injury he tried to adjust. Journalist Polly Toynbee wrote in *The Guardian*, 'He tried writing but football had been his great interest before the accident and he found he could not adapt. He was told he could never have any kind of job.' She wrote, 'He looked down at his immobilised and wasted arms and legs. "Suicide is the sensible answer for someone like me," he said. Toynbee invited the reader to agree with Haig, arguing how wrong it was that it was against the law for anyone to help Haig in his wish to kill himself: 'What Arthur Koestler could do for himself, with dignity and, one hopes, without pain, or panic, the law forced James Haig to do to himself brutishly and cruelly.' Haig set fire to his bungalow and died in the flames (*Guardian*, 25 April 1983).

Stephen Bradshaw, director of the Spinal Injuries Association and himself tetraplegic, responded to Toynbee's article. 'We are concerned that she has . . . suggested that suicide is a logical response to tetraplegia.' He could also have pointed out the inappropriate analogy which Toynbee drew between Arthur Koestler who was terminally ill and was merely choosing the form of his death which was inevitable soon, and Haig, who was not ill, who could have lived for 50 more years and whose decision was not about the form of his death but a rejection of his life.

Instead of encouraging the idea that physical disability in itself means an unacceptable quality of life, why didn't Toynbee ask why our society causes young men to think that if they can't play football then life isn't worth living? Or ask why Haig had been told he would never work again?

A liberal humanist approach to euthanasia may insist that individuals should be able to choose the manner and time of their death; that if someone genuinely feels that their life is not worth living then they should not be forced to endure pain and suffering and unhappiness. But individuals do not exist within a vacuum. We are all influenced by the values of the society in which we live. Our society not only values physical ability and perfection; it devalues and discriminates against those who do not conform to the physical norm. The prejudices against disabled people do not just exist out there in the public world, they also reside within our own heads, particularly for those of us who become disabled in adult life.

Given the level of prejudice against disabled people, we cannot realistically expect non-disabled journalists or the medical profession, or the legal profession, to mount a challenge to the assumption that a physical disability means a life not worth living. We have to challenge it ourselves. We have to question the way in which, while it is commonly assumed that a non-disabled person who is not terminally ill but who commits suicide, does so while 'the balance of their mind is disturbed', the suicide of a disabled person is often treated as rational behaviour. No mental disturbance or emotional trauma is deemed necessary to explain the rejection of life by a disabled person. Instead their physical disability is taken as sufficient grounds to want to die.

In Britain and America, disability activists have reacted with a sense of outrage at the unquestioned assumption that physical disability, *in itself*, means that life is not worth living. They have likened the acceptance that it is rational to want to kill yourself if you are physically disabled with the Nazi Euthanasia Programme of the 1930s and 1940s.

Is this an exaggerated claim? Or are there similarities between the situation today where to be severely disabled is considered reason enough to want to die, and the wholesale slaughter of disabled people which was carried out in Germany during the Third Reich?

'Unworthy Lives'

Two important books written by disabled people in the early 1980s were dedicated to the disabled people who were killed by the Third Reich. Alan Sutherland dedicates *Disabled We Stand* to 'the hundred thousand or more people with disabilities murdered by the Third Reich' and Susan Hannaford's *Living Outside Inside* is 'dedicated to my sisters and brothers, whose fate is so significant – systematically killed by the Nazis and forgotten.' Neither of the books contains any information about the mass murder of disabled people but their dedications were an illustration of the growing awareness during the 1980s among disabled people that such a slaughter had happened. In 1982 Keith Armstrong wrote about the Nazi Euthanasia Programme in an early issue of *In From the Cold* (the publication of the Liberation Network of People with Disabilities) and Richard Reiser covered the subject in an education resource book published by the Inner London

Education Authority in 1990 (Armstrong, 1982; Reiser, 1990).

While knowledge of the Holocaust is part of our general culture – as it should be – knowledge about the killing of disabled people is not. It is only in more recent years that knowledge about the other groups of people – gypsies, gay men and lesbians as well as disabled people – who were killed by the Nazis (and knowledge about the ideology and value system which motivated this killing) has started to be represented within our culture.

The recognition that, at a particular point in history, the lives of disabled people were so devalued as to necessitate our wholesale slaughter is very painful.

Robert Proctor, in his analysis of the Nazi Euthanasia Programme, *Racial Hygiene: Medicine Under the Nazis*, distinguishes between the euthanasia which is about allowing people the right to choose the time and manner of death, particularly in the case of living with pain and suffering, and the euthanasia which is motivated by a wish to relieve society of the burden of 'useless lives'. He writes:

> It is one thing to guarantee someone the right to die without suffering or without the use of heroic or extraordinary measures. It is another thing to require that certain individuals or groups be forcibly destroyed as lives useless to the community – lives not worth living. The logic in each case is different: in the first, the goal is to provide individual happiness in the final moments of life; in the second, the goal is an economic one – to relieve society of the financial burden of caring for lives considered useless to the community (R Proctor, 1988, p. 178).

Proctor's research in fact shows how the Nazi's Euthanasia Programme combined the two applications of the idea of 'mercy killing'. Both these motivations for the killing of disabled people were also apparent in the debates on the subject which took place, not just in Germany before the coming of the Nazis to power, but also in America and in Britain. In a Harvard speech in 1938, W G Lennox, while claiming that saving lives added a burden to society, argued that physicians should recognise 'the privilege of death for the congenitally mindless and for the incurable sick who wish to die'. German physicians accused after the war of having killed disabled, sick and mentally ill people, were able – with some justification – to argue that they were only putting into operation ideas which had found (and continued to find) support in other countries. In America, for example, a Gallup poll in 1937 showed that 45 per cent of the American population favoured euthanasia for 'defective infants' and in 1942 an article in the official journal of the American Psychiatric Association called for the killing of all 'retarded' children aged over five (Proctor, 1988, p. 180).

There are two crucial elements which the American 'assisted suicide' cases and the Nazi Euthanasia Programme have in common. The first is the unquestioned assumption that physical or intellectual disability, or mental illness, can in themselves be the sole, and inevitable, cause of a person's life being considered not worth living. The second is that those who feel entitled to pronounce that a life is not worth living because of disability are not disabled people themselves but non-disabled people in positions of political, economic and medical power.

There is also of course another common element – that it is not within the power of disabled people to either determine their needs for a good quality of life or to achieve the things which will make their lives worth living. It is non-disabled society which has control over financial resources, over residential establishments, over housing, personal care services, transport and all the other resources essential to achieve a good quality of life.

The Nazi Euthanasia Programme, which killed over 70 000 adults and 5 000 children during its official phase and over 200 000 in total, arose in a society which placed little value on the lives of people who were physically or learning disabled, or mentally ill. However, the Nazi idea that the lives of people with a physical or mental impairment or mental illness were not worth living was not an idea which arose out of the blue. It did not even belong solely to the Nazi ideology or to Germany.

The publication of Darwin's *Origin of Species* in 1859

was followed by the application of the principle of natural selection to human beings and society by scientists and political theorists throughout America and Europe. American social Darwinists were relatively optimistic, looking on those who survive as by definition those who are most fit. This enabled them to argue the superiority of industrial capitalism and entrepreneurial competition. German social Darwinists, however, were less optimistic about whether those people and societies that survived were necessarily the fittest, 'given the rise of revolutionary democratic movements (the French Revolution, German Social Democracy) and policies designed to secure minimum standards of welfare in the spheres of medicine and social services' (Proctor, p. 14). As Proctor points out, 'The degeneration of the race feared by German social Darwinists was said to have come about for two reasons: first, because medical care for "the weak" had begun to destroy the natural struggle for existence; and second, because the poor and misfits of the world were beginning to multiply faster than the talented and fit' (p. 15).

Social Darwinism in Germany, and in England and America, questioned the wisdom of 'medical care for the weak' on the grounds that this would encourage such people to survive and reproduce who would otherwise not survive. During and after the first world war, there was a growing fear in Germany that the 'unfit' were reproducing at a higher rate than the 'fit'. Hermann Siemens (of the Siemens industrial family) wrote in 1918 of his belief that 'care for the weak' was associated with what he called 'the proletarianisation of the population: the fear that various inferiors of the world – the poor and the weak, but also the sick and the insane – were beginning to multiply more rapidly than more "gifted" elements of society, by which was usually meant the military, political, and intellectual elite' (Proctor, pp. 18–19).

It is important to recognise that the early racial hygiene movement does not fall neatly into a left-right division.

Many racial hygienists supported a kind of state socialism whereby a strong central government would direct social policy toward programs to improve the race . . . [and conversely,] . . . Many socialists identified eugenics [encouragement, or discouragement, of reproduction according to assumptions about which social groups have desirable genes] with state planning and the rationalisation of the means of production; many thus found the idea of a 'planned genetic future' an attractive one (Proctor, p. 22).

The cross-fertilisation of ideas is apparent in the person of Alfred Grotjahn who is today considered the founder of German social medicine and one of the leading architects of Weimar Germany's progressive health reforms, and who advocated both compulsory sterilisation and increased power to commit 'defective asocials' to psychiatric institutions (p. 22).

In such a situation, the lives of disabled people in general, but particularly those of people living in institutions in Germany, were very little valued. Such people suffered especially during and after the First World War when, with the rest of the population experiencing hunger and deprivation, "defectives" were low on the list of priorities. 'As a result, nearly half of all patients in German psychiatric hospitals perished from starvation or disease' (R Proctor, 1988, p. 178).

Once the Nazis came to power in 1933, however, more definite action was taken to rid society of the burden that the institutionalised population was considered to be. The first stage of this was the sterilisation programme. In Germany, and in other industrialised countries, there was widespread acceptance that it was right to take action to prevent certain categories of people from being born. The German Law for the Prevention of Genetically Diseased Offspring was passed in 1933, but such a law had already been passed in 1907 by the American state of Indiana, the first of 29 American states to pass compulsory sterilisation laws covering people who were thought to have genetic illnesses or conditions. Other European governments which passed such laws were Denmark (in 1929), Norway (1934), Sweden (1935), Finland (1935) and Estonia (1936). In the late 1930s, Czechoslovakia, Yugoslavia, Lithuania, Latvia, Hungary and Turkey also followed suit.

About 400 000 people were compulsorily sterilised during the Third Reich. Doctors were required to register anyone known to them who had any of the 'genetic' illnesses, including 'feeble-mindedness, schizophrenia, manic-depressive insanity, genetic epilepsy, Huntington's chorea, genetic blindness or deafness, or severe alcoholism.' (Proctor, p. 96.) The sterilisation programme was largely ended in 1939, for the reason that 'the year 1939 marks the beginning of the Euthanasia Programme, in which individuals were not simply sterilised but killed' (p. 115).

Compulsory sterilisation and the ideology behind it were not confined to Nazi Germany. This was illustrated by the fact that after the war

> allied authorities were unable to classify the sterilizations as war crimes because similar laws had only recently been upheld in the United States. West German authorities thus provided compensation for persons who had been sterilized only if they could prove they had been sterilized *outside* the provisions of the 1933 Sterilization Law – that is, if they could prove they were not genetically alcoholic, epileptic, feeble-minded and so on. Compulsory sterilization ended after the war in Germany but it continued elsewhere (Proctor, p. 117).

Religion often offers powerful arguments on the sanctity of human life, and the governments of most industrial countries have to contend with their religious establishment's ability to influence public opinion. Public support for the government and for Hitler in particular was a very important part of the strength of the Third Reich. The Protestant church, the largest in Germany, generally raised no objection to the sterilisation law, and its institutions participated in the registering and recommending for sterilisation. In some cases sterilisations were also carried out in and by the church-run institutions. For example, the Bethel Mission, which cared for people with epilepsy, carried out 1093 sterilisations during the period 1934–45 (H Gallagher, 1990, p. 226).

The Catholic Church was formally opposed to sterilisation, articulated by the papal encyclical in 1930, but the German

Catholic hierarchy actually reached an agreement with Hitler that they would agree to differ on the matter (Gallagher, pp. 227–8). In any case there was disagreement within the Catholic Church, with some theologians arguing, as one Jesuit professor did, that sterilisation could be supported, 'when there were medical indications . . . that the welfare of society required such a measure or as punishment to prevent future crimes' (Quoted by Gallagher, p. 266).

Such disagreement within the Catholic Church became clear when Hitler sounded out the Catholic authorities on the question of killing people who were 'genetically defective'. At the beginning of 1939, Professor Dr Josef Mayer, who taught moral theology at the Catholic University of Paderborn, was asked to write an 'Opinion' for Hitler on the attitude of the Catholic Church towards euthanasia (G Sereny, 1977, p. 66). The paper he wrote concentrated on the mentally ill. Professor Mayer took an historical approach, arguing that whipping, torturing and burning of mentally ill people during the Middle Ages stemmed from Christ's pronouncements that they were possessed by the devil. He argued that although in more modern times a large number of theologians had rejected euthanasia for mentally ill people, this was not unanimous and that therefore an absolute moral position could not be arrived at. He concluded that 'as there were reasonable grounds and authorities both for and against it, euthanasia of the mentally ill could be considered "defensible".'

Hitler concluded 'that unanimous and unequivocal opposition from the two Churches was not to be expected and ordered the Euthanasia Programme to be started' (Sereny, p. 68).

The destruction of 'lives not worth living'

Racial hygiene ideology was based on the notion that action could and should be taken to eradicate diseases and characteristics which 'weakened' the human race. Such an ideology underpinned the policies of first isolating and then exterminating the Jewish population.

This ideology, which devalued the lives of disabled people,

became increasingly influential in determining attitudes towards disability. Within the general culture in Germany or other countries in the 1920s and 1930s there was very little positive representation of disabled people to counteract the threat to their lives. America had a president whose disability was deliberately kept completely invisible to the American and international public for fear that this disability would detract from his authority and status (Gallagher, 1985).

What representation there was of disabled people in Europe and America tended to promulgate the notion that their lives were not worth living, thus colluding with what became the dominant view within the medical profession in Germany in the 1930s. An example of this was a novel, *Sendung und Gewissen* (*Mission and Conscience*), published in Germany in 1936, which became a bestseller, about a young woman with multiple sclerosis, who decides her life is no longer worth living. Her doctor agrees to give her the means to kill her, and her husband administers the fatal morphine injection. When the doctor is charged with murder his defence is 'Would you, if you were a cripple, want to vegetate forever?' He is acquitted on the grounds that his was an act of mercy. The book was made into a very successful film.

The author of *Mission and Conscience*, Helmut Unger, was an ophthalmologist (eye specialist) who was appointed in 1939 to the newly formed Committee for the Scientific Treatment of Severe, Genetically Determined Illnesses. His task was to prepare for the killing of 'deformed and retarded children' (Proctor, p. 186).

In August 1939, this committee sent a report to all state governments in Germany asking that midwives and doctors register children born with 'congenital deformities'. By this they meant children born with 'idiocy or Mongolism (especially if associated with blindness or deafness); microcephaly or hydrocephaly of a severe or progressive nature; deformities of any kind, especially missing limbs, malformation of the head, or spina bifida; or crippling deformities such as spastics' (p. 186). Doctors who had such children aged up to three in their care were also required to register them. Payment was to be received for registration of each such child or baby.

Three members of the committee (all eminent physicians) processed the questionnaires which were returned with each registration.

Children slated to die were marked with a plus sign; children allowed to live were marked with a minus sign. Decisions were made entirely on the basis of these questionnaires; those doing the selection never examined the children in person or consulted the families or guardians.

Children marked with a plus sign were ordered into one of the twenty-eight institutions rapidly equipped with extermination facilities, including some of Germany's oldest and most highly respected hospitals . . . Parents were told that the transport was necessary to improve treatment for their child.

Methods of killing included injections of morphine, tablets and gassing with cyanide or chemical warfare agents. Children at Idstein, Kantenhof, Gorden and Eichberg were not gassed but were killed by injection; poisons were commonly administered slowly, over several days or even weeks, so that the cause of death could be disguised as pneumonia, bronchitis, or some other complication induced by the injections. Hermann Pfannmuller of the hospital at Eglfin-Haar slowly starved the children entrusted to his care until they died of 'natural causes'. This method, he boasted, was least likely to incur criticism from the foreign press or from 'the gentlemen in Switzerland' (the Red Cross). Others simply left their institutions without heat, and patients died of exposure. Nazi medical men could thus argue that their actions were not technically murder, for they were simply witholding care and 'letting nature take its course'. Parents were informed with a standardized letter, used at all institutions, that their daughter or son had died suddenly and unexpectedly of brain edema, appendicitis, or other fabricated cause; parents were also informed that, owing to the danger of an epidemic, the body had to be cremated immediately (Proctor, p. 187).

The notion of 'mercy killing' was still part of the motivation for such a programme, however. Although by the autumn of 1941, the programme had been expanded to include children up to the age of 17, it still excluded Jewish children – on the grounds that they did not deserve the 'merciful act' (p. 188). It wasn't until May 1943 that the programme was widened to include children of unwanted races and then all these children – non-disabled and healthy as well as disabled and sick children – were included.

The Committee for the Scientific Treatment of Severe, Genetically Determined Illness also set up the adult euthanasia programme in 1939. Earlier that year, authorisation had been given by Hitler to carry out the extermination of 'die Vernichtung lebensunwerten Leben' (lives not worthy of living). This authorisation was also couched in terms of 'mercy killing'. It read, 'Reichsleiter Philip Bouhler and Karl Brandt, MD, are charged with the responsibility of enlarging the authority of certain physicians to be designated by name in such a manner that persons who, according to human judgement, are incurable can, upon a most careful diagnosis of their condition of sickness, be accorded a mercy death' (Gallagher, 1990, p. 46). It was this adult Euthanasia Programme that developed the technology for mass killings which was to be used for the Holocaust. Six hospitals were equipped with gas chambers disguised as showers and cremtoria to burn the bodies.

The kind of information which was gathered about the institutional population gives an indication of who was selected for killing. All long-term hospitals, sanatoriums and asylums were circulated with questionnaires to be filled in about their patients and the accompanying instruction leaflet made clear which patients were to be registered:

All patients are to be reported who:
  1. Suffer from the following diseases and can only be employed on work of a mechanical character, such as sweeping etc., at the institution:
  schizophrenia,
  epilepsy (if not organic, state war service injury or other cause)

senile maladies

paralysis and other syphilitic disabilities refractory to therapy

imbecility, however caused

encephalitis

Huntington's chorea and other chronic diseases of the nervous system; or

2. Have been continuously confined in institutions for at least five years; or

3. Are in custody as criminally insane; or

4. Are not German citizens or not of German or related stock according to their records of race and nationality (Gallagher, 1990, p. 65–66).

The information gathered enabled the separation out of those whose disability resulted from war service. Such people were initially exempt but later on those with a mental disturbance (such as shell shock) could only be exempt if they had also been wounded or decorated for their war service. The fourth category enabled the initial exemption of non-Aryans from the programme on the grounds that 'The government did not want to grant this philanthropic act to the Jews' (quoted by Gallagher, 1990, p. 69). Later, the information gathered enabled all non-Aryans in institutions to be systematically murdered regardless of their physical or mental condition.

The authorities had a clear idea at the beginning of the programme as to how many people should be killed. They worked to the formula that for every 1,000 Germans, 10 needed some form of care, five required continuous care and, of these, one should be destroyed. This meant that their target for the adult programme was 65,000–70,000 (Proctor, p. 191). When the programme was officially halted in 1943, ostensibly because of protests from the Catholic Church and fear of public criticism, this target had in fact been reached.

However, both the adult and the children's programme continued unofficially throughout the war and in some places after the war. Three months after the end of the war the institution in the German town of Kaufbeuren was found to be routinely murdering its inmates (Proctor, pp. 192–3).

Had a wholesale 'madness' seized the medical profession and those who assisted them in this genocide? On the contrary, the killing of mentally and physically disabled children and adults was but the logical development of attitudes and theories which were deeply entrenched within the medical profession. Medical science was underpinned by general social values which threw a huge question mark over whether such lives were worth living. The assumption that they were not, combined with the application of social Darwinism in a medical context, led to the almost inevitable conclusion that for the sake of both the individual and of society, such lives should be destroyed. That genocide did not happen (at least in a planned and recognised sense) in other countries is more to do with counterbalances such as religion and the Hippocratic oath than with the absence of some kind of 'madness' which seized the German physicians. The wholesale destruction of people who were called *untermenschen* (subhuman) in Nazi Germany (Gallagher, 1990, p. 38) was a logical reaction to the medical theories, and the dominant ideology, of the time. The programme was carried out in an orderly fashion and with very little opposition.

Physicians who would not participate in the programme were not punished; neither were heads of institutions who refused to allow their patients to be taken. However, the great majority of both the medical profession and those running institutions participated in the programme without protest. Even though only a small number of physicians was directly involved with the programme, the whole profession knew about the killing of children and adults; they had to be aware as they filled out long questionnaires on their patients. 'No doctor could have been unaware of the depletion of the hospital wards or the disappearance of his patients. The doctors stood silent as their chronic patients received medical referrals to other doctors who would kill them. They did not protest – neither alone nor through the respected medical societies of Germany' (Gallagher, 1990, p. 63).

Psychiatrists seem to have been more concerned that the

sterilisation and Euthanasia Programme would put their profession out of business than with the welfare of their patients. Karl Schneider, an eminent psychiatrist, warned at the congress of psychiatrists in 1941, 'Should not eugenics, racial improvement and other measures taken by the state be able so to free the Volk from the social, moral and economic burden of the insane that psychiatry will no longer be needed at all?' (p. 63).

Franz Stangl ran one of the institutions where people were brought to be killed (and was later the commandant at Sobibor and Treblinka). His justification (after the war) of his involvement illustrates how important was the general devaluation of the lives of physically and mentally disabled people.

Stangl said that the way that the whole programme was presented to him made it seem inevitable and rational. He was told that 'it was already being done by law in America and Russia; the fact that doctors and nurses were involved; the careful examination of the patients; the concern for the feelings of the population' (Sereny, 1977, p. 52). Others however were more blatant in their denial of the right to life. Captain Christian Wirth, who was appointed as an inspector of a number of institutions, spoke of 'doing away with useless mouths' and said that 'sentimental slobber about such people made him puke' (p. 54). Wirth killed people by shooting them in the back of the head in the early days of the programme.

If people like Stangl had any doubts, they were often dispelled by the attitudes of others. Stangl paid a visit one day to an

institution for severely handicapped children run by nuns . . . When I arrived, the Mother Superior, who I had to see, was up in a ward with the priest and they took me up to see her. We talked for a moment and then she pointed to a child – well it looked like a small child – lying in a basket 'Do you know how old he is? she asked me. I said no, how old was he? 'Sixteen', she said. 'He looks like five, doesn't he? He'll never change, ever. But they rejected him.' [The nun was referring to the medical commission.] 'How could they not accept him?' she said. And the priest who stood next to her nodded fervently. 'Just look at him,' she went on. 'No good to himself or anyone else. How could they refuse to deliver him from this miserable life?' This really shook me, said Stangl, 'Here was a Catholic nun, a mother superior, and a priest. And they thought it was right. Who was I, then, to doubt what was being done?' (quoted by Sereny, p. 58).

Few people either involved in the killings or who came to know about them doubted what was being done (although there were some exceptions, such as Bishop von Galen, Pastor G Braune and the population of the village of Absberg [see Gallagher, 1990]). At his trial in Nuremberg after the war, Dr Karl Brandt, who set up the programme, made no apology for what he had done, arguing that euthanasia was justified 'out of pity for the victim and out of a desire to free the family and loved ones from a lifetime of needless sacrifice' (Gallagher, 1990, p. 257). His lawyer cited juries across the world who refused to find as guilty people who had 'freed their nearest relatives from the torment of life'. The Nuremberg War Crimes court responded to Brandt's case by saying that the issue of whether or not euthanasia was justified was not their concern. Instead what they were interested in was that, 'The evidence is conclusive that almost at the outset of the program non-German nationals were selected for euthanasia and extermination.' They concluded, 'We find that Karl Brandt was responsible for, aided and abetted, took a consenting part in, and was connected with plans and enterprises . . . in the course of which murders, brutalities, cruelties, tortures and other inhumane acts were committed [against non-German nationals]. To the extent that these criminal acts did not constitute war crimes they constituted crimes against humanity' (quoted by Gallagher, 1990, p. 259).

By insisting that the issue was the selection of non-Germans for killing, rather than the question of whether the killing of mentally and physically disabled people was justified as 'mercy killing', the court effectively avoided the essential moral issue raised by the Euthanasia Programme.

Ironically, there is considerable evidence that non-Germans were initially exempt from the programme and that their inclusion only came later when the other part of the justification for killing disabled people – namely that they weakened and polluted the Aryan race – was applied to non-Germans and to Jews.

Valuing our lives

The arguments about whether disabled people's lives are worth living, and whether the medical profession should enable us to be 'released from misery' are as threatening today as they were in the Germany of the 1930s and early 1940s. In such a context, we must insist that our lives have value. We need to question fundamentally the assumption that to be disabled, to be different, means that life is not worth living.

We are sometimes ourselves guilty of undermining the lives of disabled people. Those of us who walk with crutches often think that to have to use a wheelchair would mean life was not worth living, and those who do use a wheelchair but have the use of our arms and hands think that to be completely paralysed would be sufficient reason to commit suicide. Maybe we *would* feel like that if such a progression of disability happened, but we don't know for certain. What is more important is the fact that by assuming that a worsening of our disability means that our lives would no longer be worth living, we are undermining the lives of those who are already more disabled than ourselves.

Carol Horner is a paraplegic whose physical condition means that she may lose the use of her arms and hands in the future. She spoke at a Spinal Injuries Association (SIA) meeting about what this might mean to her.

I have chosen to live quite alone and to depend upon nobody for my personal and physical needs. I am lucky that at T6/7 [paralysis from the chest down] I was able to make that choice. This time last year, before my last operation, I decided that if it were unsuccessful and if I could no longer transfer myself from beds, chairs and loos;

and if I could no longer drive a car (a basic necessity for real independence); and if I could no longer do the things that I had had to relearn 14 years ago and if I had to rely upon others or even enter an institution for permanent assistance – then I didn't want to know. I would take steps to deliver myself from a situation that I would probably find intolerable. In other words I would commit suicide,' (SIA Newsletter, No. 25, November, 1982, p. 15).

I would support Carol Horner's right to take her own life if she should find such a situation intolerable. However, there were members of the Spinal Injuries Association listening to her speech who cannot transfer themselves without help from beds, chairs and loos, and who do not drive a car (some of them because they can't afford one). To hear that dependence on others for personal assistance means that life isn't worth living is a fundamental undermining of their lives.

We need people to value our lives, and we also must value the lives of other disabled people and refuse to make assumptions about the quality of life based on the nature of a particular disability.

Sara Johnson was diagnosed as having multiple sclerosis when she was 18. By the time she was 23, she used a wheelchair, her eyesight was affected and she needed help with feeding and dressing herself. She committed suicide and her parents, with whom she lived, were convicted of aiding and abetting her suicide. The judge, in sentencing Mr and Mrs Johnson to a year's probation gave tacit approval to the 'moral and ethical' grounds for their action but nevertheless maintained that what they did was against the law. The Voluntary Euthanasia Society publicised the case, arguing that Sara Johnson was 'incurably ill' and that her parents were carrying out a 'supreme act of compassion'.

We may feel that it *is* a compassionate act to help someone to end a life which is intolerable to them. But the danger in this case is the same as that of the American 'assisted suicide' cases, namely that there is an assumption that disability, in this case the physical condition brought about by multiple sclerosis, is *in itself* sufficient to explain the intolerable nature of the life experienced. The Voluntary Euthanasia Society (ves) argued that those who would condemn Mr and Mrs Johnson for their action

> are the people who harshly insist that incurably ill patients must see their illness through to its conclusion no matter what distress and indignity that entails. However, I am sure the sympathy of the vast majority lies with them and also with our aim to make it legal to allow medical help to die for patients such as Sara. Cases like this can only serve to strengthen our resolve to achieve this aim' (ves No. 38, January 1990).

Disabled people must demand of organisations such as the Voluntary Euthanasia Society, of the courts and of the general population, that they fundamentally question *why* a physically disabled person may find their life not worth living. To assume that the physical condition itself is the answer is to ignore the social, economic and personal context of disability. If we accept that the quality of Sara Johnson's life was *inevitably* intolerable, there is no need to put money into research on managing incontinence or other physical conditions which accompany ms. There is no need to develop housing and personal assistance services so that someone like Sara Johnson could live independently of her parents. There is no need to enable the most disabled people to get access to leisure activities. If to lose your eyesight means that your life is a write-off, what's the point in developing the technology which turns the printed word into speech?

While accepting the right of an individual to terminate their own life, we must continue to question whether their decision was right, or inevitable. Sara Johnson's decision to die should be taken as a condemnation of the services which were available to her – to do otherwise is to embark upon the line of reasoning which reaches the same conclusion that German physicians arrived at in 1939.

The British Medical Association, in its policy on euthanasia, clearly distinguishes between those who are terminally ill and those who are physically disabled. The association states that doctors should not comply with a request from physically disabled patients to be killed or to be allowed to die. The medical profession's duty, they say, is to make such a patient's life as rich and meaningful as possible. They continue

> Contemporary culture worships bodily perfection and physical pleasure. This attitude to what makes a life worth-while often dominates the thoughts of patients, friends and relatives when considering a new disability. The tra-dition of humanitarian concern in medicine is to seek values that will remain when these prejudices are removed and not to acquiesce to the shallow picture of human worth upon which these prejudices draw. It remains a tragedy that this young person is robbed of many of the joys of fully active life, but it is also a spur to find a creative, not a destructive response to that tragedy (British Medical Association, 1988, p. 45).

As disabled people we need to encourage positive attitudes towards the value of our lives, not only among the medical profession, but also among those whose social, economic and political power can influence all the other things which have a far greater impact on the quality of our lives than does our disability itself.

In an article in *Social Work Today*, Chris Heginbotham (then Director of MIND), claimed that 'no one is seriously suggesting that voluntary euthanasia should be allowed for healthy individuals . . . but only for those with terminal ill-nesses, a poor prognosis and the likelihood of extreme pain or distress in those final few hours or days.' For disabled people the situation is not so simple. The idea that disability means that our lives are not worth living is so powerful that it creeps into both medical (despite the BMA's statement) and moral judgements.

Ruth Moore, one of the women I interviewed, has been told that her spine is crumbling at the level at which she may be unable to breathe unaided and would have to use a respirator. The risk of becoming completely paralysed is very great. The non-disabled world already tends to judge that her current level of physical disability must mean a quality of life that would be unacceptable to them. Ruth is very worried about the kind of attitudes that the medical profession brings to the situation of someone like her when her physical condition deteriorates.

> The neurosurgeon told me that he was only interested in quality of life and that in no way would he be looking to prolong my life if he didn't feel the quality would be acceptable. However, neither he nor anyone else has asked me what criteria *I* would use in judging what was an acceptable quality of life. I am very worried that if I get admitted unconscious or without the power of speech, he will take a decision based on *his* judgement and *his* criteria about what is an acceptable quality of life.

The prejudice and ignorance which are widespread among people who can have a major impact on not just how we live our lives, but whether we live at all, can be frightening. We have to establish our own values about our lives and insist that non-disabled people recognise such values.

As Barbara Waxman, an American disability activist, said,

> I don't think society understands anything about disability. People look at me and they ask me how do I live my life. I think what they're really asking is *why* do I live my life? They believe that the pain that I experience is derived from my functional limitations. What they don't understand is that the pain and rejection I've experienced have been purely socially based. I'm not depressed about being disabled. I'm quite skilled at being a disabled person. I'm quite proud of my identity as a disabled person. But the pain is social (Waxman, 1990).

Barbara Waxman also identified the way in which the assumption that our lives are intolerable, and costly, dominates the development of genetic screening, the debates on abortion and the issue of 'allowing' disabled babies to die.

> This is a time when disabled people are coming out more and more and voicing the pain and the struggle which is derived, not from having a disability, but from the preju-

dice and the social rejection and the political and economic discrimination which we experience. And rather than taking responsibility for assisting in transforming both the built and social environments which will accommodate disabled people they are using science to cure what *they* determine the problems to be.

These are the issues which lie at the heart of the next chapter.

Chapter 3:
The Chance of Life

Were I a foetus doomed to disablement I would be eternally grateful to a doctor who released me from the dreadful life inflicted upon me – letter read out on BBC Radio 4's PM programme.

I didn't want to write this chapter, because it meant facing my own disablism. It also meant asking some very hard questions about feminism's failure to take into account the interests of disabled people.

During the 1970s – before I became disabled – I was involved in all the campaigns to defend the 1967 Abortion Act. 'A woman's right to choose' seemed so central a demand to countering women's social and economic oppression and it was outrageous that a male-dominated parliament, and a male-dominated church, should have so much power over whether women could have control over their own bodies.

Like most other feminists at that time, when defending women's right to abortion, I unthinkingly bracketed together two circumstances of unwanted pregnancy; that following rape and those pregnancies where pre-natal diagnosis found that the foetus was 'handicapped'. While feminists believed that women in any circumstances should be able to choose to end an unwanted pregnancy, we felt we were on stronger ground in arguing for abortion in these two situations as there was a wider base of public support for allowing a woman to refuse to carry either a rapist's child or a 'handicapped' child.

However, in 1983 I became disabled and I spent the rest of the decade reluctantly realising that I had been part of a movement which, by promulgating such arguments, contributed to disabled people's experience of prejudice and oppression.

Abortion on demand

The fourth demand of the Women's Movement in Britain is 'Free contraception and abortion on demand'. When this demand was formulated in 1970 it was seen as central to achieving social, economic, political and personal equality. In modern capitalist societies, the situation in which most women have children – the nuclear family – is the location of women's oppression. Having children makes women dependent on either men or the state because they are expected to provide unpaid child-care and this limits their economic activity. Feminists argued that women's liberation would come out of 'the struggle for a total change in the economic, work and family structure of society. But this freedom to struggle will not come about until we have control over our own bodies' (M Sjöö, 1972, p. 188).

Having a child has significant social and economic consequences for women, and the importance of the ability to say no to the powerlessness which too often comes with being a mother should not be underestimated. The demand that women, rather than the medical profession, should have the right to choose whether to continue with a pregnancy, is an assertion of our control over our own bodies. The 1967 Abortion Act still left the decision in the hands of doctors, but it at least legalised abortion under certain conditions.

If motherhood generally is associated with dependency and powerlessness, motherhood where the child is physically or learning disabled is even more likely to result in a situation where an individual woman is struggling to care for a child in a social and economic situation characterised by powerlessness. The privatisation of childcare within nuclear families has significant consequences for women (and their children) when a child has the greater physical and emotional care needs often associated with disability and where those needs may continue beyond childhood. Most women in such situations find that the support offered to them to care for their child at home is inadequate and many find that the only alternative is unsatisfactory residential care for the child.

Almost all women who choose to have an abortion, for whatever reason, find it a painful decision. However, for many it is also a fundamentally liberating decision; it is an issue of control over one's life and body and therefore to be able to choose is to be empowered.

Disability activists (who, of course, include disabled feminists) may recognise that the ability to terminate an unwanted pregnancy is an important part of women's ability to take control over their lives. However, for most non-disabled women, the discovery that a foetus has a physical or learning disability will, in itself, transform a wanted pregnancy into an unwanted pregnancy. This is the source of conflict between a disability rights perspective on abortion and a feminist perspective. Now that I am physically disabled, I feel hurt and outraged at the judgement that physical or learning disability can turn a welcome for a new life into a denial of life.

The factors involved in turning a wanted pregnancy into an unwanted one in these circumstances are complex. Disabled people have argued that when a woman decides to abort a disabled foetus, she is not so much choosing as being constrained to take such a decision. Faced with the knowledge that her child will be physically or learning disabled, the message she will generally receive from the medical profession is that disability is an expensive tragedy. She will certainly be aware that to bring up a disabled child is a struggle given the inadequate resources that society makes available. She is also likely to bring her own prejudices about disabled people to the decision.

Most feminists engaged in the abortion debate have done little more than acknowledge these points and have made few attempts to confront the prejudice which lies at the heart of their assumption that disability is a justification for abortion. Because of feminism's failure to incorporate the interests of disabled people, disability activists have been faced with the unenviable choice of either being aligned with the anti-abortionist organisations such as the Society for the

Protection of the Unborn Child (SPUC) and LIFE; or supporting 'a woman's right to choose' but feeling extremely
uncomfortable that such an alignment with non-disabled feminists has meant supporting a woman's right to abortion
merely on the grounds of disability.

The abortion debate has intensified in recent years following medical advances in pre-natal screening. Developments
in ultrasound have increased the identification of physical
abnormalities in the heart and spinal cord during the first
five months of pregnancy. Research on genes has enabled the
detection of particular physical and intellectual conditions in
the early stages of pregnancy.

At the same time, medical advances have meant that
babies born prematurely are surviving at earlier stages of
gestation and this has given more strength to the anti-abortionists' arguments that to terminate a pregnancy is to kill a
human life. In Britain, during the late 1980s some anti-
abortionists, such as the MP David Alton, adopted the tactic
of trying to lower the time-limit at which abortions could
legally be carried out.

This tactic was finally successful in 1990 when an amend-
ment was successfully made to legislation going through parliament on human embryo research. This had the effect of
introducing a new time limit of 24 weeks for all abortions
except when either the foetus was 'seriously handicapped',
when the mother's life was at risk, or when there was a risk
of permanent injury to her if the pregnancy continued. This
new time limit came about primarily because of increasing
support within the medical profession for a reduction in the
28 week limit imposed by the 1929 Infant Life (Preservation)
Act. It was now clear that 24 weeks' gestation was the point
at which a baby could survive. However, both the medical
profession and the majority of MPs and members of the House
of Lords wanted to enable women to terminate a pregnancy
where prenatal diagnosis (often only possible at 22–24 weeks)
indicated disability. The effect of the legislation is that, if a
foetus has been diagnosed as having a physical or learning
disability, termination of the pregnancy is now legal right up
until the moment of birth.

During parliamentary debates on this issue, those arguing

in favour of exempting women carrying disabled babies from the new time limit argued that the quality of life of such babies and children was intolerable, that the burden imposed on their parents was insupportable and that they constituted a high economic and social cost. Amendments which would have given the medical profession a duty to preserve a life after 24 weeks' gestation – i.e. when the foetus has a viable life outside its mother's body – were outvoted. As John Habgood, Archbishop of York, who does not normally ally himself with the anti-abortionists, pointed out, the new legislation means that 'seriously handicapped people may be destroyed simply because they are seriously handicapped' (House of Lords Official Report, 18 October 1990, Col. 1049).

Non-disabled feminists have generally failed to confront the judgements about disabled people which are an integral part of this debate. Feminism itself is the poorer for this, as I will argue. Before doing this, however, it is important to recognise that feminism is also the poorer for failing to take on board the links which disabled people have made between the arguments about abortion and disability and the issues around 'allowing' disabled babies to die.

One British case where a disabled baby was 'allowed' to die resulted in the prosecution of Dr Leonard Arthur in 1981. He was accused of murdering John Pearson, a Down's syndrome baby. As the baby had been rejected by his parents, Dr Arthur had instructed that he should be 'given nursing care only'. This meant that he was sedated and given no milk. The baby died within three days. The judge at his trial referred to Dr Arthur as a 'caring and compassionate man' and called Down's syndrome people 'walking time bombs of infection and disease' (a singularly ignorant and offensive remark). Dr Arthur was acquitted.

During the course of the public debate on whether the baby should have been allowed to die, a disabled woman, Micheline Mason wrote 'I do not want to discuss the issue. You are speaking about my life. You wish me to discuss whether or not, as a woman born with a "severe" disability, I think I should have been murdered. It does not sound reactionary to me to hear of people who want to put an end to the killing of babies because they have disabilities. It sounds wonderful' (M Mason, 1982a).

All three of the arguments which have been part of the debate on abortion and disability were at play in this incident. First, the judge and the doctor assumed that the baby's quality of life would be intolerable; second, the parents had felt the child would entail high personal costs for them. Last, the judge gave voice to the assumption that such a child constituted a drain on society's resources. I want to look at these arguments in turn.

Quality of life

Arguments about the potential quality of life for a disabled child take place in the context of a society which is generally hostile towards disabled people. Feminism has let disabled people down by failing to confront these 'quality of life' arguments.

As a society we cannot, and should not, make judgements about the quality of other people's lives (or of potential lives). When we react to the disability of others, or the prospect of disability in a child, we bring our own subjective experience to the situation. Any assessment of whether someone else's life is worth living can only be based on what their life means to us, not on what it means to them. To give ourselves the right to judge someone else's life as not worth living – based on the assumption that we *can* make such a judgement – is to enter the same ideological framework as the German physicians in the Third Reich, for it is important to recognise that 'mercy killing', was a key motivation for their wholesale slaughter of disabled people. Our society does not allow our medical profession to exercise such a policy in respects of adults who become disabled. Neither should we allow the medical profession to make judgements about the potential quality of life for an unborn child. Such judgements can only take place in the context of our society's prejudice against disabled people.

In making judgements about the quality of our lives, non-disabled feminists and the non-disabled world in general have fundamentally undermined the value of our lives and our right to exist. In failing to examine their own preconceptions and ignorance about living with a disability, non-disabled feminists have created an inevitable conflict between a feminist and a disability rights perspective and this has harmed both political movements.

However, it is also important to recognise the way in which the disability movement has often been thrown onto the defensive in the attempt to assert the value of our lives. In asserting our right to exist, we have sometimes been forced into the position of maintaining that the experience of disability is totally determined by socio-economic factors and thus deny, or play down, the personal reality of disability. It is difficult to integrate this reality in a positive way into our sense of self when the non-disabled world has nothing but negative reactions to the physical and intellectual characteristics of disability. In this way, an assertion of our worth becomes tied up with a denial of our bodies and an attempt to 'overcome' the difficulties which are part of being disabled. We can thus fall into the trap of trying to prove that our lives are worth living by denying that disability sometimes involves being ill, in pain, dying or generally experiencing a bloody awful time.

One of the strengths of feminism has been to give voice to personal experiences. The domination by men of the disability movement has been associated with an avoidance of recognising our feelings about being disabled. A feminist perspective on disability must focus, not just on the socio-economic and ideological dimensions of our oppression, but also on what it feels like to be unable to walk, to be in pain, to be incontinent, to have fits, to be unable to converse, to be blind or deaf, to have an intellectual ability which is much below the average. There are positive and strong elements to these experiences but there are also negative and painful elements. The tendency of the disability movement to deny the difficult physical, emotional and intellectual experiences that are sometimes part of the experience of disability is a denial of 'weakness', of illness, of old age and death.

While the negative parts to the experience of being Black or gay in a white, heterosexist society can be identified as wholly socially created, there are negative aspects of being disabled which would persist regardless of the kind of society in which we live. We should not be made to feel that we have to deny these negative things in order to assert that our lives have value. For myself, I feel that even if the physical environment in which I live posed no physical barriers, I would still rather walk than not be able to walk. However non-discriminatory the society in which I lived, to be able to walk would give me more choices and experiences than not being able to walk. This is, however, quite definitely, *not* to say that my life is not worth living, nor is it to deny that very positive things have happened in my life *because* I became disabled. I can therefore value my disability, while not denying the difficulties associated with it.

We need courage to say that there *are* awful things about being disabled, as well as the positive things in which we take pride. If we feel strong enough to do this, we can truly challenge the way non-disabled people make judgements about our lives because in so doing we will take charge of the way in which disability is defined and perceived. Unfortunately, the tendency of the disability movement to avoid giving expression to how we feel about being disabled means that non-disabled people have only their own feelings about disability to influence them.

In order that our lives can be seen in a balanced way, we must demand the right to be heard when we assert that there are wonderful things about being disabled. But we must also demand that it is we who define the negative things about the experience – and not the medical profession, health and social services professionals, parents or other non-disabled people. And in the context of abortion, we must not allow judgements about the potential quality of life for an unborn disabled child to enter into the debate about whether or not a woman should have an abortion. Our society must recognise that each individual can only judge his or her own life and not that of others.

It is not for us to judge whether another human being's life is worth living. Neither is it for the medical profession to exercise such judgements. When the British Medical Association faced the question of euthanasia for disabled adults, they recognised the pressures resulting from prejudice. In rejecting 'mercy killing' for such people they said, 'The tradition of humanitarian concern in medicine is to seek values that will remain when these prejudices are removed and not to acquiesce to the shallow picture of human worth upon which these prejudices draw' (BMA, 1988, p. 45). Unfortunately, when the BMA, in the same publication, faced the issue of 'allowing' disabled babies to die, they failed to make such an unequivocal statement. Yet this philosophy should be applied to both babies and to unborn babies – whether before or after conception. Each of us is only qualified to judge the quality of our own life.

In fact the 'quality of life' arguments, in the context of preventing disabled children being born or surviving, are often something of a smokescreen for the more important motivations involved; that is, when neither society nor individuals as parents are prepared to take on what are perceived to be social, economic and personal costs involved in having a disabled child.

A woman's right to choose?

Where a woman whose foetus has been diagnosed as disabled decides to seek an abortion, or a woman asks a doctor to 'allow' her disabled baby to die, she is saying that she does not wish to take on the social, economic and personal costs of having a disabled child. In order to determine whether we think we can support a woman's right to so choose we need to look at a number of factors involved.

First, there is the nature of the choice being made. When arguing for abortion rights, the women's movement has found it tactically productive to emphasise women's rights as individuals and to appeal to the liberal humanist tradition within Europe and America. However, the emphasis on the rights of women as individuals has tended to obscure the constraints within which choices are made. As Sue Himmelweit wrote in an important article published in *Feminist Review*,

Reproductive decisions, like all others, are always made within a material and cultural context. To see it as the context providing the options and the individual making the choice is only one way to look at such a situation: the one favoured by liberal ideology . . . The context may be better seen as constraining, ruling out what might appear to be alternative courses of action, even at times to the point of effective determination (S Himmelweit, 1988, p. 42).

It is significant, Himmelweit points out, that women facing the decision about whether to abort a disabled child often talked about the decision they made – whichever one it was – as their only choice. She says, 'This contradictory phrase sums up neatly the problem with the notion of freedom of choice in situations where one action is undertaken only to avoid even more dreadful alternatives. The emphasis such women would put is on the lack, not the availability, of choice that the combination of their social and medical conditions imposes on them' (p. 42).

The most important constraints within which women 'choose' whether or not to have a disabled child are the knowledge that society does not provide adequate resources for disabled people and the ignorance and prejudices which they, in common with most non-disabled people, hold about disability. Similar socio-economic and ideological constraints operate when women in India 'choose' to abort female foetuses following amniocentesis or when women in China 'allow' their newborn daughters to die (p. 41, 45). In both countries the social and economic disadvantages of being female, and the prejudice which is associated with this, are strong enough to pressurise some women into avoiding giving birth to daughters.

Another problem with appealing to the rights of the individual in supporting the right of a woman to choose not to bear a disabled child is that, in giving her such a right, the individualist tradition also tends to place the responsibility for action solely on the individual, with a concomitant denial of social or collective responsibility. Such a denial is manifestly against both the interests of women and of disabled people. Both groups, because of their lack of power in the marketplace, need a society which recognises collective responsibility for those who are economically less powerful.

If the responsibility is placed on the individual woman to exercise the choice over whether or not to give birth to a disabled child, then the responsibility for choosing to bring up such a child also rests on her. As Himmelweit says, 'We may find that resources, instead of becoming more abundant because fewer such babies are born, are cut on the grounds that women had the right to choose not to bear such a child' (p. 43). Certainly, one of the consequences of genetic screening (where a couple can be screened before conception for the risk of some hereditary conditions), prenatal screening and abortion is that women are pressurised into 'choosing' not to have a disabled child; for example, a study published in 1985 found that a majority of doctors would only offer amniocentesis to women if they agree in advance to have a termination if the foetus is 'abnormal' (Wendy Farrant, 1985).

The second factor which we have to consider in relationship to a woman's right to choose an abortion is the rights of the unborn child. In the 1970s, the attacks on the 1967 Abortion Act and attempts to rescind or undermine it were very much couched in terms of the status of the foetus as a human being. The Catholic Church teaches that life begins at the moment of conception and that any human action to end that life is therefore murder. In their attempts to counter this argument, which was seen as treating women as mere reproductive machines without considering their rights as human beings, feminists were forced into denying that the unborn child has any human status. As Himmelweit writes, 'Basing the claim for access to abortion on women's individual rights has forced feminists to maintain a hopelessly insensitive position on the status of the foetus, dismissing it as just a "clump of tissue" or a "bunch of cells" (p. 50).

Most women who have abortions do not in fact feel like this about the foetus growing inside them, and certainly women who have late abortions – as most abortions on the grounds of disability are – are taking a decision to end a life which has usually become very real to them. Feminists have tended to shy away from the recognition of the foetus as having the status of a human being because of the association of this argument with anti-abortion organisations such as SPUC and LIFE. Yet Wendy Savage who, as Himmelweit says, 'could not have more respectable feminist credentials on the abortion issue', states, 'I have always agreed with the anti-abortionists that life begins at conception, that a new individual starts at conception and that doing an abortion is not the same as removing an appendix because you have got this other potential person there.' She poses the issue in terms of a balance of conflicting rights between mother and child: 'As the foetus becomes larger, its rights become greater, and there comes a point . . . where the foetus's right to live equals the right to get the pregnancy terminated' (quoted by Himmelweit, p. 50).

It is important that we face up to the fact that aborting a foetus of 8 weeks' gestation is not the same as aborting one of 24 weeks' gestation. The fact that a baby born at 24 weeks can now survive (because of recent developments in neonatal care) *is* an important factor in what women, doctors and nurses feel about terminating such a pregnancy. This is *not* to say that in no circumstances should a pregnancy be terminated after 24 weeks. It is, however, to recognise that another human being is involved and that the rights of the mother and the rights of the child may be in conflict. Furthermore, if we accept the arguments which I have made about the quality of life we must also maintain that the same rules should apply to disabled foetuses as apply to non-disabled foetuses. It is outrageous that, under legislation just passed in Britain, a foetus of more than 24 weeks gestation is treated as having rights as a human being but loses these rights once it is diagnosed as being disabled.

If we accept that the more advanced the pregnancy the more rights the potential child has, then we certainly have to accept that a child who has already been born also has rights. This issue has been much debated by American disabled feminists in the context of what are known as 'Baby Doe' cases. In these situations, as a group of American disabled feminists write,

the infant is born with a severe disability and needs medical attention to survive. If given, the medical treatment will prolong the life of the child, but it will not lessen the child's disability. An example is that of an infant with Down's Syndrome. She or he has a permanent mental impairment that may range from mild to severe. Let us say that shortly after birth the infant develops a blood infection and needs medical treatment to save its life. But the treatment, which may be very expensive, will not lessen the infant's mental impairment. These parents decide they would rather withhold treatment, thus pitting their right to privacy in making decisions regarding the welfare of their child against the right of the disabled child to live. Part of the parents' rationale for withholding medical treatment relies on the telethon 'disability as tragedy' theory.

Applied in this context, that argument says that a disabled infant imposes such an emotional and financial burden on the family that the state has no right to prohibit the parents from relieving themselves of the burden. Viewed from the parents' perspective, the argument appears compelling; take away the blinders imposed by the 'disability as tragedy' theory, however, and the Baby Doe issue becomes a clear-cut case of civil rights. Viewed from a civil rights context, a disabled infant should not receive a different standard of medical care solely because of her or his disability. If a non-disabled infant developed a blood infection, there would be no question of a right to life-sustaining medical treatment (Blackwell-Stratton *et al*, 1988 p. 317).

Do we want to live in a society where judgements made about other people's (potential) quality of life result in differential medical treatment and a removal of the protection of the law against murder? We are not dealing here with the issues which arise when someone is terminally ill and experiencing a level of pain which makes them feel their life is not worth living. Instead we are talking about other people deciding that physical or intellectual difference means that life is not worth living. I have already argued that we should have the humility to say that we cannot judge the quality of another's life. Neither should we give parents the right to decide whether their child lives or dies. Such parents may well decide that they cannot take on the social, economic and personal costs of a disabled child, but to say that this abdication of responsibility should result in the child's death is to support the politics of individualism to inhumane conclusions.

The question of collective responsibility leads us to consider the final motivation for preventing disabled children being born or surviving.

Social and economic costs of disability

As medical technology develops, babies, children and adults who previously would have died survive and sometimes their survival is seen as costly in economic terms. The Department of Health promotes screening for spina bifida on grounds of the 'large demands' that spina bifida children and adults make on the health and social services (Davis, 1990, p. ix); Peter Thurnham MP declared during the course of a House of Commons debate on abortion in 1985 that to abort a 'handicapped' foetus could well save the country £1 million over the course of a lifetime.

It is undoubtedly true that disability can have high economic costs – costs which would be even higher if adequate resources were devoted to ensuring a good quality of life. It is also the case, however, that a society which did not disable people with a physical or intellectual difference would instead enable such people to make a significant social and economic contribution. Furthermore, it is the distribution of resources which is more important. We need to ask whether, for example, weapons of destruction are a more acceptable subject of public expenditure than developing the technology and services which make life tolerable for one group of people. As Micheline Mason writes, 'There are enough resources to support everyone in a comfortable, fulfilled life, whether they live in London and have spina bifida, or live in Bangladesh and are starving. It is the big illusion of our time that it is the resources that we lack. The problem is some people control them, misuse them, and deny them to the majority of the rest of the world' (Mason, 1982a p. 26).

It is also important to consider whether the prevention of disability involves costs in itself, either to disabled people or to society generally. For example, the Spinal Injuries Association is involved in educating schoolchildren about the dangers of certain physical activities such as diving (a cause of spinal cord injury). The way that this is done does not undermine the lives of people with spinal cord injury because the SIA is careful to promote positive images of disabled people and at the same time is involved in campaigning for adequate medical and rehabilitation services for people who incur a spinal cord injury. There is no discernible cost therefore to either society or disabled people of taking this preventive action and the benefits are clear.

At the other end of the scale is, say, the case of a child born with Down's syndrome, whose parents reject him and where the medical profession feels able to take action which will lead to his death (this action would be either sedation and a withholding of sustenance as in the Dr Leonard Arthur case, or a withholding of medical intervention necessary to save the child's life). 'Allowing' such a child to die may save society economic resources but permitting such a practice incurs other costs. It creates a situation where the medical profession has the right to judge whether someone should live or die, on the basis of their assessment of the quality of that person's life. This gives a power to the medical profession of which we should be very wary. We are not willing to give it this power in respect of adults and, if we accept the argument that a baby or a viable foetus has rights as a human being, then we should not give the medical profession power over their life or death either.

Such practices are also a denial of collective responsibility and a buttressing of individual responsibility. Doctors take such decisions when parents reject a disabled baby. The principle operating is therefore that if the parents as individuals do not take responsibility for such a child then society will refuse to take collective responsibility. The disability movement argues that society should make adequate resources available for those whose physical and intellectual differences mean that they have particular needs. In so doing we maintain that this is our right as citizens and that a society which seeks to be humane and just should recognise and celebrate diversity. It is difficult to do this if societal values at the same time advocate the termination of the lives of babies whose needs are different from the norm.

Most importantly, a situation is created which undermines the value of the lives of those people with Down's syndrome who already exist. As I have argued above, we have no right to judge the quality of other people's lives and to recognise this is to recognise a fundamental civil rights issue for disabled people. If the preferred course of action is to prevent Down's syndrome babies surviving (or, indeed, being born) this undermines the financing of research and development on living with Down's syndrome, and the provision of services to enhance the quality of life.

By condoning the killing of another human being – whether this is a baby born at full term or a 'viable foetus' – we are placing an enormous emotional burden on those involved. In 1988 a doctor wrote (under the pseudonym 'Ivy Walker') of something she had done 16 years earlier and how the resulting guilt and sorrow had stayed with her since. As a paediatrician she had been called to deal with an anencephalitic (brainless) child who had been born alive but was not expected to live for more than a few hours. The parents had been told that the child would be stillborn and the hospital had wanted to spare them the anguish of having to register the birth and then the death of the child. Professional thinking on allowing parents to grieve over the death of a new-born child has since changed but at the time it was thought best that the child was treated as a stillbirth. Dr Walker wrote,

> But the baby, a girl, was not dead. I stood in the sluice, among the sterilisers and bedpans, wondering how much longer she could go on breathing. Apart from the entire absence of brain, she was perfect in every other way. The obstetric staff came in and out of the sluice, more distressed at every visit. They were adamant that the baby must not live, even for a few hours, as that would mean

the parents would have to be told she was alive . . . It was
made clear that I was the paediatrician and the baby was
my problem. At the time, I also believed that the parents
should be saved more anguish. So I turned the baby on
her face, put a pillow over her head and held it there until
she stopped breathing.

It took 20 minutes for her to die. They were the longest
20 minutes in my life. I became increasingly distressed and
when eventually she did die, I fled the maternity unit in
tears. I do not know what happened to the baby's body
afterwards, though I suspect it was taken to the hospital
incinerator because the whole point of the exercise had
been to ensure there was nothing for the parents to have
to bury.

. . . It was very wrong of us to deny those parents the
opportunity to grieve. We probably prolonged the very
distress we were trying to prevent. Hardest of all to live
with is the knowledge that I caused another human being
more distress in death than she would have had dying
naturally. This baby would certainly have died within a
few hours – why, why did I have to interfere? (I Walker,
1988).

She provides the answer to this question herself when she
states that, 'The baby herself, because of her handicap and
closeness to death, was not part of the equation, was not
considered a human being'. The costs involved in taking such
an attitude were not just those of greater suffering for the
child but also greater suffering for the parents and an
emotional burden for the doctor which she will carry for the
rest of her life.

In all situations where someone is treated as less than a
human being, the costs are high for the perpetrators of this
action as well as for the recipient. If we devalue human life
we become less human ourselves.

A feminist and disability rights perspective

We need to combine both a feminist and a disability rights
perspective on the issues of screening (both before and

during pregnancy), abortion and 'allowing' disabled babies to die. Some disabled feminists have reacted to the dilemma posed by non-disabled women choosing to abort disabled foetuses by saying that they support such women's right to choose, while wishing that they wouldn't choose to deny existence to a disabled child. But this is avoiding the issue.

There is no absolute right to choose whether to have a disabled child or not. An acceptance of such an absolute right belongs within an individualist tradition which, in the last analysis, gives all rights and responsibilities to individuals with no recognition of the collective rights and responsibilities of society. It is not in the interests of either women or disabled people to rely on liberal individualism for the furtherance of our rights.

With respect to genetic screening, disabled people quite rightly feel that the prevention of particular disabilities undermines the existence of those living with that disability. But we would be foolish to take the view that genetic screening to prevent a particular condition is never justified. For example, a woman faced with the knowledge that her unborn child has Lesch-Nyhan syndrome – a very rare condition in which the child develops a compulsive tendency to bite off their own fingers and tongue – may well feel that it would be cruel to allow the child to be born.

However, whether and how we support genetic screening has to be determined by the other costs involved balanced against the benefit of preventing some level of suffering. The Afro-Caribbean community, for example, may legitimately argue that to fail to put resources into enabling children to be born without the risk of sickle-cell anaemia (an hereditary blood condition which particulary affects Black people and which can be painful, physically limiting and shorten lives) is to discriminate against the Black community. On the other hand, if the cost of such resources is compulsory screening and the prevention of those with sickle-cell trait from having children, then such preventive action is unacceptable. Jewish communities have good historical reasons to be wary of genetic screening because of its potential use for eugenicist purposes. However, such communities may also feel that to fail to develop preventive action in the case of Tay-Sachs disease (which causes blindness, learning disability and early death and which is found in Jewish communities of Eastern European origin) would be to cause unnecessary hardship.

These examples indicate the complexities of the issue. It is however, important to state – unequivocally – that the widespread assumption that the prevention of disability through genetic screening is a legitimate goal throws into question our right to exist. Women whose disabilities have a genetic origin also have much to fear from the development of genetic screening within current societal values, as there is likely to be great pressure on them not to have children. Ironically, although non-disabled feminists have failed in the past to take on our concerns, feminists such as Hilary Rose have more recently identified that there is a danger that the new reproductive technologies – from genetic screening to test tube babies – are developing in ways which are coercive of women in general (H Rose, 1987). Surely there is scope here for a feminist and disability rights perspective on genetic screening which addresses the interests of both women and disabled people?

In the case of abortion, since in our society the major costs of having a disabled child fall on individual women, it is only right that women should have some power to determine whether or not to terminate a pregnancy where the child is discovered to be disabled. How much power they should have, however, has to be balanced against the extent to which the foetus has rights as a human being. I would argue than once a foetus, disabled or non-disabled, has a viable life outside its mother's body, its rights as a human being are greater than its mother's right to refuse to give birth to it. The option still remains, of course, for the mother to refuse to care for the child, but in that case it is society which must take on the responsibility; we should accept collective responsibility and accept the rights of the baby as a human being.

In the case of doctors taking action, or failing to take action, which results in a baby's death, none of the motivations put forward to justify such action are valid. It is not for us, or the medical profession, to judge the quality (or potential quality) of someone's life on the basis of their physical or intellectual characteristics. We can do nothing other than bring our own subjective judgements – and fear of disability – to an assessment of a disabled baby's potential quality of life.

The second motivation which I discussed – the opinion held by some parents that bringing up a disabled child will impose an intolerable burden on their lives – is a justification for parents (and particularly for mothers as they will be the most affected) to refuse to care for such a child. But this should not undermine the collective responsibility for accepting such babies as human beings and doing everything possible to enhance the quality of their lives. Moreover, the negative effects of killing disabled babies or children on the kind of society we live in, and the effect on the individuals concerned, far outweigh the economic costs of such children's survival.

A reliance on individualism to further our interests – as women or as disabled people – in the final analysis does nothing more than bolster the same type of values that lie at the heart of the social Darwinism which I discussed in the previous chapter. Individualism refuses to recognise interdependence and collective responsibility, relying instead on the survival of the fittest to bring about a healthy, efficient society. In such a society there would be no room for the kind of choice which Marsha Saxton, a disabled feminist, wants to make. 'At this point, if I became aware that the foetus I was carrying would be disabled, I would not choose to abort it. These are my reasons. I hope for and look forward to a time when all children can be welcomed to a world without oppression. I would like to exercise this view if only in my own personal world' (M Saxton, 1984).

This chapter, and the previous one, have dealt with situations where our very existence is at risk. The devaluation of disabled people permeates the general culture, often in more subtle ways, and this is the subject of the next chapter.

Chapter 4:
Disability in Western Culture

This chapter looks as the representation of disability within Western culture. By this, I mean the messages, images and ideas about disabled people which are contained in all the different forms which reflect and promote Western culture. I am not attempting a systematic analysis of the portrayal of disability in specific cultural forms; rather I am seeking to reflect on the way that the general culture portrays our lives. The chapter draws heavily on critiques which have already been made of the cultural representation of disability by disabled people themselves. Such work is also part of the creation of a disability culture and is a crucial part of our self-liberation.

Where am I – as a disabled woman – in the general culture that surrounds me? Generally, I am not there. I could watch television for years, possibly a lifetime, without seeing my experience reflected in its dramas, documentaries, news stories. I could spend a lifetime going to theatres, libraries, bookshops, reading newspapers, without finding any portrayal of a disabled woman's life which speaks to my experience. I can try to affirm my existence by watching the 'specialist' disability television programmes, produced by disabled people but squeezed into tiny, out-of-peak-viewing-time slots. I may discover one or two books (if I'm *very* lucky) in my local feminist bookshop which reflect my reality. Apart from this, if I want to maintain my confidence in the validity of my experience, I must steadfastly ignore the portrayal or lack of portrayal of disabled people within the general culture. Otherwise, I may come to believe that the non-disabled world's definition of me and my life is the real one – and my reality is mere fantasy.

The general culture invalidates me both by ignoring me and by its particular representations of disability. Disabled people are missing from mainstream culture. When we do appear, it is in specialised forms – from charity telethons to plays about an individual struck down by tragedy – which impose the non-disabled world's definitions on us and our experience. However, that is the situation within the general culture (and also the feminist culture which similarly ignores or misrepresents disabled women's experiences). Outside of the general, and the feminist, culture there is an emerging disability culture, without which I would not be able to write this book. Elspeth Morrison, a disabled woman involved in promoting disability arts, writes, 'Disability Arts and Disability Culture are relatively new terms. They are an acknowledgement by a growing number of disabled people of our common heritage, shared experiences and most important of all, our common oppressions' (E Morrison, 1989).

Sian Vasey, who has also done much to promote a disability culture, argues that we need to create 'our own body of artistic work about or informed by the experience of being disabled in the same way as there is already much work created from the point of view of women, people from ethnic minority cultures and from lesbians and gay men' (Sian Vasey, 1989). 'Ultimately,' she writes, 'disability culture should be recognised as one of the many strands running through contemporary multi-cultural society.'

The way that the general culture either ignores or misrepresents our experience is part of our oppression. However, mainstream culture is also the poorer for this. Surely, the representation and exploration of human experience is incomplete as long as disability is either missing from or misrepresented in all the forms that cultural representation takes. It is fear and denial of the fraility, vulnerability, mortality and *arbitrariness* of human experience that deters us from confronting such realities. Fear and denial prompt the isolation of those who are disabled, ill or old as 'other', as 'not like us'.

The kind of experience explored in the poem 'The Wolf' is very frightening. It is written by Susan Hansell, a woman writer who has Lupus, a chronic illness which 'causes my immune system to make antibodies against my own DNA; this means my body is literally devouring itself'. Many people would prefer to flee from the pain of her reality. But from this reality Susan Hansell has created a powerful representation of something which is part of human experience.

[The Wolf]

I

i write
    when it hurts

last night i dreamt
   there were tubes in my back
my body
      hooked
   to machines,
this morning i couldn't bend over

i write
    when it hurts

last night
i dreamt
   the soles of my feet split
i walked on bare bones
     glass splinters grinding in my joints

i write
    when it hurts

my mind pouring out through my fingertips
     relieved
my body melting into images i create
       relieved
the words
   tie me
     to a past
   to a future
     where our lives are re/lived
over and over

write it down   write it all down

push
the pencil
across
the page

i write
    when it hurts

searching for words
        to tell
            how it feels

II

in a dream i am walking alone at night   i come to an
intersection of wide streets   and stop to peer in every
direction   i am very careful   i begin to cross   then
a car drives speeding heading right for me   i can't run
i can't run away   i'm not able to run

somehow   i jump onto the hood   this life still in me
i curse   make fists   and pound against the windshield
but there is no one to hear me   there is no one driving

i wake
  to the cries of a wolf
circling
    my brain

my mind spins
  into the day while
        my body lags behind
licking
            the wounded legs
    the swollen joints

if
the pain controlled me
i might
tear through my flesh and pull open the back bones
spine by spine

if time controlled me
i might never sleep
    there's so much left
undone

but i have learned the power of each breath
in and out

III

i dream i have 10 days to live
i flee the city for the earth's edge
      where the water turns mountains to sand
  and lie naked
     under yellow cliffs
       spilling
   salty currents
        into the sea

rivers run from my pores
  until i float
on my own
    dusty bones

  will you
       take me
     take me

  turn my body
   into smooth round stones
        and scatter me
     across
      the shore

(Susan Hansell, 1985.)

If the experiences of disabled people are missing from the general culture this means that non-disabled people have few points of reference with which to make sense of our reality. Furthermore, the tools which they *do* have to interpret our experiences are those fashioned by non-disabled people. This can have significant consequences for our lives, particularly because we so rarely have the power to insist on the validity of our experience. It can mean that we are denied the basic human rights that non-disabled people take for granted; it can also mean that our experience is denied and this can have devastating consequences.

The denial of our reality can result in the kind of oppression experienced by Edwina Franchild. She has retinitis pigmentosa, 'a condition that caused me to have tunnel vision, night blindness, sensitivity to bright light, and slow adjustment to changes in light' (E Franchild, 1985, p. 37). This condition was not properly diagnosed when she was a child and she was subjected to a range of physical and emotional abuse as a result of the failure of the adults around her (professionals as well as her family) to recognise and accept the way that her eyes worked.

She writes:

Eventually, while I continued to believe that there was something indefinably wrong with me, I grew to understand that there was also something wrong with the way I was being treated. Some deep part of me must have known it was wrong to be humiliated and punished for something that was a natural and unchangeable part of my being. As parents, grandparents, teachers and ophthalmologists conferred about possible ways to 'help' me, I began to sense the presence of a plot. Since I did not fit the acceptable category of 'sighted' or even the less acceptable but still comprehensible category of 'blind', I threw those who came into contact with me into confusion. I was a creature who existed between two concepts, and they strove hard to get me to fit into one or the other. 'Blind' meant helplessness, irrationality, hopelessness, darkness, even an association with death itself. 'Sighted' meant hope, rationality, capability, life. Given these choices, the adults around me tried to force me into the sighted mold. They did this partly by taking me to eye doctors who might be able to 'cure' me, but mostly by simply denying that I could be anything but sighted.

Edwina's family insisted that 'She just sees what she wants

to see'; a teacher asserted that 'She'll see better and better as she learns to use her eyes' and her father told her this over and over again.

> Thus, the whole reality of my experience was being denied, and I was told that it did not exist. Part of me believed that I must be crazy and deficient to perceive things so differently than they did. But an older pre-language part of myself realised that they were trying to deny my existence and therefore my life itself. *They were trying to kill me.* I then hypothesized that there was a world-wide conspiracy that was trying to do away with me, for some completely unfathomable reason. This feeling of mine was expressed by fear of and endless rage at my parents; I had frequent tantrums and kept running away from home. My parents and the school authorities decided I was deeply disturbed; I was sent in now for a new round of testing: psychological. I was given every test imaginable, including a brain scan, to see if my brain was damaged. I was taken in for counselling at a 'child guidance' center. When that did not seem to work my parents committed me to a state psychiatric hospital for children. The year was 1962 and I was ten years old (pp. 38–39).

The failure of the adult world to recognise Edwina's sight as a natural and unchangeable part of her being arose from two cultural reactions to physical limitations. The first is the 'wrongness' of physical limitation or difference, thus the parents' desire for their child to be 'alright'. The second is the stereotyping of physical limitation even when it is recognised. Edwina's parents would have been better able to recognise total blindness as a legitimate experience – that is, an actual physical experience – because there is a cultural stereotype of the blind person and this stereotype gives meaning to an otherwise incomprehensible experience (albeit a distorted meaning).

However, because Edwina's physical characteristics did not fit neatly into this stereotype, her experience was invalidated – and thus her very identity undermined. The adult world then interpreted her reaction to the way they treated her as pathological. Yet in actuality, the child's reaction to the adults' behaviour was utterly rational and reasonable. They were threatening her very existence; the adults around her were all-powerful – to her they controlled the entire world as she knew it – and, for reasons which she could not begin to understand, they were acting in ways which would destroy her.

We all experience oppression as a result of the denial of our reality. If our reality is not reflected in the general culture, how can we assert our rights? If non-disabled people would rather not recognise disability, or only recognise specific forms, how can they recognise our experience of our bodies? If we do not 'appear' as real people, with the need for love, affection, friendship, and the right to a good quality of life, how can non-disabled people give any meaning to our lives?

Our values and our ways of looking at our experiences – if they are freed from the way that the non-disabled world defines us – are an important part of the diversity of human experience. However, non-disabled people's feelings about our differences often make our attempts to take our place within that culture difficult and painful.

Our attempts to 'come out' as not normal and to explore the pain, as well as the joys, of our existence, are often either ignored by the non-disabled world or evoke uncomfortable feelings which people find difficult to confront and therefore find it easier to ignore. A *Time Out* review of 'One in Ten', a photographic exhibition of disabled people going about their daily lives, concluded, 'The motive is honourable, but pictures of deformed people are horrifying and set up a chain of unpleasant reactions. One comes away sickened and feeling guilty about one's own responses – maybe this, in itself, is a good reason to stage the exhibition' (*Time Out*, 6 February 1981). The glimmer of insight contained in this last sentence is, however, usually snuffed out; non-disabled people are reluctant to examine their own feelings about disability in any of the cultural forms open to them. Instead, disabled people either do not appear or our lives are misrepresented and transformed into the stereotypes with which non-disabled people feel more comfortable.

The failure of non-disabled people to deal with their feelings about disability means that our attempts to represent ourselves within the general culture often become distorted or suppressed by the fear and abhorrence that disability evokes.

The meaning of disability in the general culture

It is often said that disabled men and women do not conform to the stereotypes of physical attractiveness. To be a disabled man is to fail to measure up to the general culture's definition of masculinity as strength; to be a disabled woman is to fail to measure up to the definition of femininity as pretty passivity. Just as white skin is presented as the norm – in the sense of being both the average and the goal to be strived for – so lack of physical and learning 'impairment' is also the norm.

In an important sense, the non-disabled world defines physical and learning disability by their absence. To be considered beautiful is to give value to the absence of physical 'impairment'. This is the case even in the classic stereotype of the 'beautiful blind girl', for the recognition of her beauty is equivocal, conditional. Otherwise, what would be the relevance of her blindness?

Status and authority are also associated with an absence of disability. A person who is revered cannot be disabled, for this would be to detract, to take away, from his (or less often, her) appeal. The clearest illustration of this was the American president, Franklin D Roosevelt. Roosevelt was completely paralysed from the waist down yet this was hidden from the American and international public. His aides, his family and the press, went to enormous lengths to hide his disability, the automatic assumption being that a politician who then became president of the USA must not be seen to be weak and dependent. In particular, the public never saw him in a wheelchair for this was/is the ultimate symbol of dependency and lack of autonomy (Gallagher, 1985).

But there is much more to the cultural representation of disability than the way in which the norm is measured by the absence of disability. The way in which the culture interprets and uses the *presence* of disability is the very powerful other side of the coin. Just as beauty – and goodness – are defined by the absence of disability, so ugliness – and evil – are defined by its presence.

Writers over many years, in a number of different genres, have used physical and learning disability, and mental illness, to signify evil, badness, a state of something wrong. There are obvious examples of this: from Shakespeare's Richard III to Doris Lessing's *The Fifth Child* (which uses learning disability to transmit a profound sense of threat and unease); from Captain Hook to *The Phantom of the Opera*.

The crucial thing about these cultural representations of disability is that they say nothing about the lives of disabled people but everything about the attitudes of non-disabled people towards disability. Disability is used as a metaphor, as a code, for the message that the non-disabled writer wishes to get across, in the same way that 'beauty' is used. In doing this, the writer draws on the prejudice, ignorance and fear that generally exist towards disabled people, knowing that to portray a character with a humped back, with a missing leg, with facial scars, will evoke certain feelings in the reader or audience. The more disability is used as a metaphor for evil, or just to induce a sense of unease, the more the cultural stereotype is confirmed.

In recent years, disability, and in particular disabled men, have also been used in a more complex way as a metaphor for dependency and lack of autonomy.

Masculinity and physical disability

The social definition of masculinity is inextricably bound up with a celebration of strength, of perfect bodies. At the same time, to be masculine is to be not vulnerable. It is also linked to a celebration of youth and of taking bodily functions for granted. The BBC film *Tumbledown* about a soldier injured in the Falklands war (inadvertently) exposed the cultural representation of ability and disability. 'I hate cripples, I always have,' said the hero, in his frustration at his dependence on wheelchair and crutches. The army had promised him physical strength and perfection (and authority), not the ignominy of being told off by a ward sister for being stupid enough to leave hospital while still seriously ill. His anger was part of his denial of his bodily frailty and vulnerability – and who was a mere woman to try to remind him of it?

The absence of physical 'impairment' is so clearly bound up with popular culture's images of masculinity that film makers are able to use visible physical disability as a clear statement about a character. In the past, the most common statement has been about evil and wickedness; children's and adult fiction alike abound with bad men whose sinister threat is signified by a physical difference. More recently, film makers have used disability as a metaphor for dependency and vulnerability and as a vehicle for exploring such experiences for men.

Two films, both released in 1990, had disabled men as their central characters and received much publicity for the way that they supposedly dealt with the reality of disability. *My Left Foot* was a British film based on the autobiography of writer and artist, Christy Brown, who had cerebral palsy, while *Born on the Fourth of July* was an American film based on the true story of a Vietnam soldier, Ron Kovic, and portrayed his experience on returning home paralysed.

In fact, rather than being about disability, both these films, as critic Judith Williamson writes, are actually about how awful it is for a man to be dependent, in the emotional sense as much as the physical. 'These films are about the hell of dependency for men. And maybe the men have to be in wheelchairs for that dependency to be made vivid.' The films rely on the general association of impotence with disability, and on the association of heterosexuality with a stereotyped masculinity.

'The strongest dynamic in these movies is the sense of sheer horror, for men, in being deprived of autonomy' (J Williamson, 1990). This is heightened by both actors, Tom Cruise and Daniel Day Lewis, being, as Williamson puts it, 'world-famous sexy pin-ups'. She goes on, 'What the image of disability does in these films is to take to breaking point the pain felt in situations not exclusive to disablement. Each man loses a lover (common enough) but the devastation and helplessness that ensue enter a whole different emotional register when they're compounded with humiliation ('not being a man'). This gives great insight into what it is to be a man, disabled or not.' In *Born on the Fourth of July*, the character played by Tom Cruise has to confront not only the appalling lack of resources to meet the needs of those who returned from the Vietnam War permanently disabled, but also the fear that his physical disability will destroy his relationships with others. Judith Williamson writes, 'After "dead penis", Cruise's next scream is, "Who's gonna love me?" Worse than feeling unloved is feeling unlovable; which is precisely what the wheelchair seems to explain.'

Daniel Day Lewis's portrayal of Christy Brown's cerebral palsy in *My Left Foot* never moves beyond using disability as a metaphor for dependency. The story is little more than the traditional 'overcoming all odds' portrayal of disability (indeed Christy Brown himself called his autobiography, on which the film is based, 'my plucky little cripple story'). The film is based on two expressions of non-disabled people's prejudice against disabled people. The first is the reaction to Christy Brown painting and writing with his left foot. The wonder at what he produced is not an appreciation of his writing or his art but rather a wonder that it is done at all.

The second expression of prejudice is a deeply patronising attitude towards Brown's love for a woman and his reaction to her announcement that she is marrying someone else. This was the scene which most reviewers of the film focused on, making much of Brown's drunken expression of anger. At a formal dinner in a restaurant, Christy Brown abuses the woman who has just told him she loves someone else, shouting and pulling the tablecloth off the table. In other words, he behaves in an oppressive, aggressive and intimidating manner, not an unusual thing for a non-disabled man to do but film critics seemed to think it was amazing for a disabled man to behave in this way. Somehow, it was supposed to be 'progressive' that a disabled man was portrayed as behaving in a thoroughly obnoxious way.

The makers of these films are not actually portraying the lives of disabled individuals; rather the disability is a vehicle for exploring the pain of dependency and vulnerability for

men. A man in a wheelchair is an easily recognisable metaphor for a lack of autonomy, because this is how the general
culture perceives disabled people. It may also be the safest
way for men to explore their vulnerability, for they can
separate themselves quite easily from the disabled character,
who is clearly 'different' from the 'normal' man. The films
do not challenge the stereotype; they use it and in so doing
exploit us.

The emotions explored in both *Born on the Fourth of July*
and *My Left Foot* are dependent on the stereotype that to
be a man in a wheelchair is to be impotent, unable to be a
(hetero)sexual being, and therefore not a 'complete' man.
The link between heterosexuality and what it is to be a man
is also crucial to the American film made in 1978, *Coming
Home*, which, like *Born on the Fourth of July*, was also
concerned with some of the issues raised by the Vietnam
War.

However, *Coming Home* was very different in that the
stereotype of disability is challenged in a fundamental way.
Luke Martin (played by Jon Voight) may be paralysed but
Sally (Jane Fonda) enjoys going to bed with him. Luke may
be physically paralysed but it is Sally's husband Bob's
emotional paralysis which is more disabling – both to their
marriage and to himself. (Bob eventually commits suicide.)
Luke holds the moral high ground. He is able to confront
not only that the Vietnam War was wrong, but that what he
did as a soldier was wrong. Bob, on the other hand, finds
this too painful to live with; he cannot imagine a role for
himself once the framework which created his role as an All-
American hero is challenged.

Coming Home was a fundamentally subversive film. It
wasn't only an anti-Vietnam War film but it also challenged
American male and female stereotypes. Luke Martin had
more to offer as a real person than the upright and uptight
Bob. The crossing over of Sally from a frigid, rigid, pillar of
the WASP community to the kind of emotional reality that
Luke represented was a triumph for a set of values which
runs counter to the Great American Dream. In this sense,
Luke's paralysis symbolised the positive alternative.

Coming Home is an exceptional film in that the daily

details of life with paralysis are shown as an integral part of a real, powerful, autonomous person. However, as with *My Left Foot* and *Born on the Fourth of July*, it is impossible to imagine a woman in the role of the disabled character. It is impossible because essentially all three films are not about disability but about masculinity; they are vehicles for the exploration of stereotyped views on what it is to be a (heterosexual) man.

Femininity and disability

As part of a research project carried out in 1986, some American college students were asked to write down whatever came to mind when they heard the phrase 'disabled woman'. Many students left their paper blank, having been unable to think of anything when they heard the term. Of those who did write something the majority wrote words signifying passivity, weakness or dependency, They wrote 'almost lifeless', 'pity', 'lonely', 'crippled', 'wheelchair', 'grey', 'old' and 'sorry' (*Disability Rag*, Jan/Feb, 1987, p 11). The exercise was part of a research project on disabled women and the researchers were surprised at the results, even though they had been expecting negative images. When the 145 students were asked to list what came to mind when they heard the word 'woman', they wrote down terms associated with heterosexuality and heterosexual relationships, work, and motherhood, These terms were almost entirely missing from the associations with the words 'disabled woman'.

Physical or learning disability in a woman has been used in the various cultural media in the same way as it has in men to signify evil or horror. But the overwhelming association with disability for women, as these students' reactions show, is one of passivity, dependency and deprivation. Even a feminist writer such as Marilyn French has used disability to signify dependency. In her novel *The Bleeding Heart*, French explores the conflicts between autonomy and dependency, strength and passivity, which many women experience within heterosexual relationships, As Deborah Kent points out, in her analysis of the portrayal of disabled women in literature,

French uses the character of Edith (who is paralysed after a car crash) to portray 'the passive, subjugated woman whom according to French, men secretly desire . . . Edith is submissive and asexual . . . [she] embodies many of the most debilitating stereotypes behind which disabled women lose their individual identities. When she loses the ability to walk, she also is robbed of her sexuality, her intellect and her sense of self' (D Kent, 1988, p. 101). In contrast, Dolores, with whom Edith's husband has a love affair, is autonomous, strong, alive and sexual. As a disabled feminist, I feel betrayed by Marilyn French's exploitation of the cultural stereotype of disability, for she is doing nothing to challenge oppressive attitudes and everything to collude with them.

Interestingly, film-makers in the 1970s and 1980s have not been as interested in the use of disability as a vehicle for exploring dependency and vulnerability in women as they have for exploring the same issue about men. There seems to be no complexity to a woman's dependency – at least not for the men who make films. Older films – such as *Whatever Happened to Baby Jane* in which Blanche Hudson (played by Joan Crawford) is 'confined' to a wheelchair and is at the mercy of her murderous sister, and *Wait Until Dark* in which Audrey Hepburn plays Susy Hendrix, a terrorised blind woman – use physical disability as a fairly straightforward representation of vulnerability. The intention is to create fear, and the audience is drawn into a sense of helplessness caused by the disability (although Hepburn's character then uses her ability to 'see' in the dark to turn the tables on her aggressor).

Generally, however, women do not have to be portrayed as disabled in order to present an image of vulnerability and dependency. Not surprisingly, therefore, most disabled characters in film and television in recent years have been men. The most common representation of disability in television and the cinema is a wheelchair user because the wheelchair offers the most obvious and easiest way of presenting a recognisable disability. Most of the disabled people depicted in this way are men. Lauri Klobas looked at 100 fictional examples of wheelchair users in film and television and found that over four out of five were men – and the great majority were white (L Klobas, p.190).

One example of a woman's disability being used in a metaphorical sense other than to represent evil or horror or dependency, was in the 1986 film version of *Children of a Lesser God* directed by Randa Haines. The stage play had been very positively received by the Deaf community because its main character, Sarah, was a strong Deaf woman who was part of a Deaf community, and who demanded that her interests and concerns be addressed by the hearing community. The story is based on the relationship between the Deaf community in a school for Deaf young people and the hearing world that surrounds them. It is also about Sarah's relationship with a hearing teacher. In the play, Sarah's strength is set within a background of other strong Deaf characters, and her struggle for her rights, including her insistence that she wants to have Deaf children, has an authority and coherence to it.

In the film, however, there are no other strong Deaf characters and Sarah's behaviour is made to seem eccentric and little more than temper tantrums. As other disabled people pointed out when the film was released, Sarah's deafness has been turned into a metaphor for the lack of communication between men and women. Mary Jane Owen wrote, 'It's a beautiful film about a beautiful couple in a beautiful landscape trying to overcome some problems they just happen to have in communication. Oh yes, she is deaf, but that's not the real problem in the director's mind. The problem's that she stubbornly refuses to recognise what's best for her' (M J Owen, 1987, p.21).

As with the cultural representation of disabled men, films such as *Children of a Lesser God* say more about what disability means to non-disabled people than anything about our real lives and concerns.

Susan Browne, Debra Connors and Nanci Stern identify two stereotypes which are frequently projected onto disabled women. 'One is the happy, humble woman who has "accepted her handicap" and is endlessly grateful for the help of others. Her counterpart is embittered, blames everyone else for her situation, and continually lashes out. Society approves of our complacency and discounts our anger. Either way, we are made invisible' (Browne, Connors and Stern, 1985, p. 77).

Disabled women particularly object to the way that there is no room for our anger because it can only be interpreted as individual bitterness. This is fundamentally undermining, As Dai Thompson writes,

> Anger felt by women because of our disabilities is rarely accepted in women's communities, or anywhere else for that matter. Disabled or not, most of us grew up with media images depicting pathetic little 'cripple' children on various telethons or blind beggars with caps in hand ('handicap') or 'brave' war heroes limping back to a home where they were promptly forgotten. Such individuals' anger was never seen, and still rarely is. Instead of acknowledging the basic humanity of our often-powerful emotions, able-bodied persons tend to view us either as helpless things to be pitied or as Super-Crips, gallantly fighting to overcome insurmountable odds. Such attitudes display a bizarre two-tiered mindset: it is horrible beyond imagination to be disabled, but disabled people with guts can, if they only try hard enough, make themselves almost 'normal'. The absurdity of such all-or-nothing images is obvious. So, too, is the damage these images do to disabled people by robbing us of our sense of reality (D Thompson, 1985, p. 78).

Some of this is echoed by Marsha Saxton and Florence Howe when they write, 'Disabled women are typically regarded by the culture at two extremes: on the one hand, our lives are thought to be pitiful, full of pain, the result of senseless tragedy; on the other hand, we are seen as inspirational beings, nearly raised to sainthood by those who perceive our suffering with awe' (Saxton and Howe, 1988, p. 105).

However, the Super-Crip role poses problems for women because it requires self-confidence and assertion and is much easier to achieve with economic security. It is not surprising therefore that most 'overcoming all odds' stories concern disabled men, although a few of such stories are about women such as Helen Keller.

Overcoming all odds

A crucial element in this type of cultural representation of disability is a striving competitiveness. This goes together with an emphasis on the individual. Within this perspective, it is not society which disables someone by its reactions to limitations and difference but the individual who either fails to 'rise above' their misfortune or who exhibits the personal strength and willpower to achieve 'against all odds'.

Christy Brown's autobiography, *My Left Foot*, and the film made from it, falls into this type of cultural representation of disability. The non-disabled world wonders at the ability of someone who has a significant speech impediment and who can only move his left foot, to paint, to write, because these are things that normal human beings do and Christy Brown is treated as fundamentally alien to normal humanity.

In the 'overcoming all odds' model of disability, the disabled person is often presented in terms of a 'brilliant mind in a crippled body', a phrase actually applied to Professor Stephen Hawking who has a motor neurone disease. The non-disabled world finds disability, or injury, difficult to confront or to understand. Other people's pain is always frightening, primarily because people want to deny that it could happen to them. Lack of control over one's body is also very frightening, particularly as it can mean such dependence on others. 'Overcoming' stories have the important role of lessening the fear that disability holds for non-disabled people. They also have the role of assuring the non-disabled world that normal is right, to be desired and aspired to.

As Pam Evans told me, 'The status quo likes us to be seen "fighting back", to resent and bewail the fact that we can no longer do things in their way. The more energy and time we spend on over-achieving and compensatory activity that imitates as closely as possible "normal" standards, the more people are reassured that "normal" equals right. If we succumb to their temptations they will reward us with their admiration and praise. At first sight this will seem preferable to their pity or being written off as an invalid. But all we will achieve is the status of a performing sea lion and not (re)admittance to their ranks.'

It is easy to be seduced into the role of being exceptional, of being 'wonderful', particularly as this is often the only (seemingly) positive role open to us. We can insist that people react to us as individuals and not as someone who is blind, or paralysed, or deaf, or learning disabled. The Spastics Society, for example, thought that they were being progressive by producing advertisements which encouraged people to look beyond the wheelchair and see the real person. But if people are being asked to ignore our disability they are being asked to deny a fundamental part of our identity and our experience.

The 'overcoming' model of disability separates us from other disabled people; it isolates us and in any case offers no more than a very conditional acceptance. Rachel Cartwright discovered this as she grew older as a blind woman:

> I spent most of my life proving that I could do everything that a sighted woman could do. I did well at school, got a reasonably paid job, got married, had children and now I have grandchildren. All that time, I pretended that being blind didn't really matter, that it was an inconvenience and that if I let my personality shine through people would treat me as anyone else. I was very successful at it. But now I'm old and what am I supposed to do about that? I can't 'overcome' being old. I could be exceptional as a blind woman, talented, develop other abilities. But as an old blind woman, there's no positive role on offer.

The non-disabled person as rescuer

Lauri Klobas, who writes about disability images, has identified that a common theme in films and television about disabled people is the portrayal of a non-disabled person as the wise, strong person who acts as a catalyst for a disabled person 'coming to terms with their disability' (Klobas, 1987, p. 192). In this type of representation of disability, the disabled person has personal and emotional inadequacies, most commonly portrayed as anger and bitterness, and/or a failure to face up to disablement. As Klobas writes, 'Attitudinal and physical barriers seldom confront these angry, bitter people'; instead the problems of disability are personal problems, related to individual inadequacies.

An example of this is the play by Tom Kempinski, *Duet for One*, about a violinist who has multiple sclerosis. The play is worth a detailed analysis because it is a powerful cultural representation of both women's dependency and the dependency of disability.

There are only two characters in the play, Stephanie Abrahams, an eminent violin player who has multiple sclerosis, and Dr Feldmann, a psychiatrist. Dr Feldmann is probably best described by the phrase used in the playwright's character notes as having an 'air of comforting wisdom'. Stephanie is a more complicated character – 'she had to rebel to realise her dream of becoming a musician, which has made her outspoken, often aggressive, witty, bitter and sarcastic sometimes, and seemingly confident. She has courage, now stretched to its limit with the knowledge that she has multiple sclerosis and knows her worth as an artist. Underneath she is, of course, in despair.'

Stephanie can still walk, although she uses an electric wheelchair to come to Dr Feldmann's office, but she can no longer play the violin and has therefore had to give up her career. She has apparently decided to find purpose in her life by acting as a secretary to her husband, who is a world-famous conductor, and by teaching the violin. It is her husband's idea that she comes to see Dr Feldmann – 'I came because my husband thought I was fairly upset with things and might benefit from some kind of, I don't know, support or guidance, and I agreed with him.'

The essence of Dr Feldmann's role is that he is an expert about Stephanie's feelings. He is even portrayed as an expert – more expert than she – on multiple sclerosis, in a swift exchange in the early part of the play. His expertise on her feelings – his authority about what she feels and what should be done about it – takes the form firstly of prescribing drugs which are presented as necessary to her emotional, and physical, survival (Feldmann immediately reveals her vulnerability to suicide), and secondly, of stripping away the surface of what she says to reveal the pain and distress she feels which emanate from her childhood experiences. 'I think it is very important for you to discover your true feelings about your position at this moment,' he tells her. And he is the source of the discovery of these true feelings.

Stephanie begins her sessions with Dr Feldmann by talking of superficialities, of presenting a positive picture of 'coming to terms with' her illness, of adjusting by becoming a teacher and her husband's secretary instead of the world-famous soloist she once was. Feldmann cuts through all this, asking her whether – since music was so important to her marital relationship – she is now afraid that her husband may leave her. In response to his skills, we learn about her childhood and its significance to her current situation. He unpeels the layers of self-deception like an onion, revealing the anger, terror and despair underneath, and the pinnacle of his expertise is achieved when she finally expresses what it means to no longer be able to make music. 'Music,' she says, 'is the purest expression of humanity that there is,' and as she confronts her loss she admits that 'you can't change this condition with determination.'

Having broken down her defences and revealed the true despair underneath, Feldmann now has the task of rescuing her, both from the very real threat of her suicide and from the nothingness of chronic depression. He describes her condition to her and sets out the goal to be achieved: 'As primitive man was the subject of the blind forces of nature, so you too are at the mercy of the dark forces of your unconscious mind; at the moment they have you in their power; you sit around, you complain, you say you can do nothing. But as that primitive man set about transforming his hostile forces to his own purposes, so you too must now engage yourself in a life activity, to master your dark forces. To succeed will be a great labour; but succeed you can and must.'

But Stephanie isn't ready yet truly to confront her loss; he has to shout at her, telling her to 'get off your arse and fight!' It is in the final scene – having in the previous week obviously done as he instructs, working on her 'inner themes and chords and progressions' – that she finally strips down to her real emotional self. 'The violin isn't my work; it isn't a way of life. It's where I live,' she says. It had become her world when her childhood world disintegrated after her mother's death. 'Everything went when she died, everything, all the normal things, everything I was used to, all the bits and pieces of ordinary life went down the black hole with Mummy . . . So I hung on to the only world I had: music. My violin. And I sang the song of the pain and the sorrow and loss and the awful changes, to soothe myself. And I sang for dear life – literally for life, 'cos it was all I had.'

Feldmann has enabled her to see what her disability means to her. And the closing line is his assertion, through his question, 'Is the same time next week still convenient?' that he can bring her back to life from the death that her inability to make music means to her.

The play is very powerful, not least because it reflects not just the loss which is sometimes an integral part of having a condition such as multiple sclerosis, but also how the nature of that loss is determined by what went before rather than by the condition itself. The problem for disabled people, however, is that Stephanie is defined, determined and rescued by a good, strong, wise non-disabled person. She cannot find the strength from within herself even to recognise and confront her loss without Feldmann's help, let alone find the ability to deal with it and live. As a woman, and as a disabled woman, Stephanie can have no true autonomy as a human being; her very survival depends on a male expert's knowledge of herself and the alternative he has to offer her. Although the play deals in real emotions, in the final analysis it merely colludes in and confirms the stereotype of the despairing, dependent disabled woman.

Not worth living

In *Whose Life Is It Anyway?*, a play by Brian Clark, the main character, Ken Harrison, *does* have autonomy – at least the play is about his struggle (which is eventually successful) to exert control over his life. Instead of the male expert holding the key to the truth, as in *Duet for One*, in this play it is the disabled man who reveals the true state of things to the female doctor. The irony is that, in the exercising of his autonomy, Ken Harrison is arguing that someone who is severely disabled cannot have a quality of life which is worth living.

Ken Harrison is a sculptor who is paralysed from the neck down as a result of a road accident. At the opening of the play he has been in hospital for some months and is expected to move soon to a long-stay hospital where he will remain for the rest of his life. The hospital has done all it can for him physically; his life-span may be a long one despite his paralysis. The doctors' response to his anger and frustration with his situation is to give him Valium, forcibly by injection when he refuses to take tablets. Ken's own response to his situation is to decide that his life is not worth living and to take legal action to exert his right to die.

A hospital orderly (who is the only character in the play who is spontaneously sympathetic and understanding of Ken's perspective) asserts that it is crazy to keep him alive at the cost of hundreds of pounds a week when in Africa children die of measles for the want of a few pounds. Ken himself has a number of reasons for wanting to die. Partly, it is because he is told he will be dependent on nursing care for the rest of his life, partly because he cannot sculpt any more, but also because he says he is not 'a man' any more.

Perhaps the most tortuous thing for him is that he feels tremendous sexual desire for Dr Scott, a junior hospital doctor, but, he says, 'I've only a piece of knotted string between my legs,' and her behaviour towards him is not that of a woman towards a man.

'It's surprising,' he remarks of her behaviour when in his room, 'how relaxed a woman can become when she is not in the presence of a man.' To Ken, paralysis has robbed him of what his masculinity meant to him, and he is thereby robbed of what he defines as his humanity. Life has nothing left to offer him.

Dr Scott initially offers the standard response to his wish to die; she says that such a feeling is common in the early stages of a high level of paralysis but that he will 'get over that feeling'. To her it would be morally wrong to agree that he should be allowed to die. However, after the exchange between them when he makes clear his sexual desire for her and the way that his inability to do anything about it means that he is no longer 'a man', Dr Scott confides to the ward sister about Ken's wish to die and says, 'It's just a calm, rational decision.'

Ken hires a solicitor to take legal action on his behalf to enable him to leave hospital, in the knowledge that in the consultant's opinion he is 'incapable of living outside the hospital' and would die. The consultant, unlike Dr Scott, remains of the opinion that Ken is suffering from depression and is 'incapable of making a rational decision about his life and death'. The solicitor calls in a psychiatrist, who judges that Ken's mind is not 'unbalanced' and that he is quite 'sane'. The solicitor then issues a writ of *habeas corpus* which would enable Ken to be discharged out of the hospital and the case is heard before a judge in Ken's hospital room. The psychiatrist attests that, by wishing to die, Ken is 'reacting in a perfectly rational way to a very bad situation'.

When the judge questions him, Ken insists that it is not that he wishes to die but that he is dead already – 'I cannot accept this condition constitutes life in any real sense at all . . . I find the hospital's persistent effort to maintain this shadow of life an indignity, and it's inhumane'.

The judge concludes, 'I am satisfied that Mr Harrison is a brave and cool man who is in complete control of his mental faculties and I shall therefore make an order for him to be set free.'

This play – which was made into a very successful film starring Richard Dreyfus – merely gives voice to the way that the non-disabled world generally reacts to disability. The notion that our lives are not worth living is so deeply rooted and unchallenged that the play can present Ken Harrison's wish to die as a struggle of an individual against a bureaucracy (as represented by the hospital consultant). In fact, the play is really about the non-disabled world's definition of disability.

Charity

There is one cultural context in which disabled people are very much present – although grossly misrepresented. This is the use by charities of images of disability in their fund-raising activities. The role of charities and the cultural representation of disabled people on which they rely constitute a fundamental undermining of disabled people as autonomous human beings; as Ruth Hill argues, charities create a culture of dependency (R Hill, 1990). We are recipients of other people's goodwill. As such we are essentially passive in that it is in the power of others to determine whether we are a deserving case. At the same time, our gratitude is an essential part of the relationship; charity is actually about making the non-disabled person feel good about themselves. Our gratitude is the gift we are expected to make in exchange for tolerance and material help.

Material help from charities is dependent on the charities' definitions of what constitutes a 'deserving case' and this undermines our rights to the things which make a reasonable quality of life possible. Although charities collect money from the general population, they very rarely give disabled people money; this would be to give us too much power. Instead the help is in the form of equipment, holidays, and so on. Health and social services professionals play a key role in defining what we need.

The images and messages that charities propagate about the lives of disabled people also create a culture of dependency. Charities need to present disability in such a way as to encourage people to part with their money. The portrayal of a strong disabled person going about his/her life, and enjoying it, is not going to bring in any money. It isn't so much that negative images are necessary in order to raise money. As one advertising agency said, 'Negative imagery won't get us what we want . . . but if you portray people running happily and successfully and having fun, it can have a negative effect [on the success of the advertisement in raising money]. People need to see there's hope, but you can push success too far' (Susan Scott-Parker, 1989, p.9).

It is an emotional reaction which charities are seeking, and the emotions which provoke people to give money are those of pity and of guilt. People need to be stirred by the plight of an individual or a group of individuals; they feel genuine pain at the sorrow which is presented to them and are made to feel that they must do something to help. In such a situation, giving money is easy and it eases the pain which the image has evoked.

Images of disabled people are also used to make people feel that they are lucky; to feel relief that their life, their child, is not like that. But this sense of relief can bring a sense of guilt (which is often experienced only as a sense of unease). Again, it is easy to soothe this reaction by giving money.

Charities occupy a particularly significant role in the cultural representation of disabled people because, as organisations, they are seen to be synonymous with the group of disabled people that they purport to represent. The interests of people with cerebral palsy are assumed to be represented by the Spastics Society, of those with muscular dystrophy by the Muscular Dystrophy Group, and so on. As a study of advertising and disabled people put it, 'Charities tend to commission [advertising] campaigns as though they owned their particular "model" of disabled person, in much the same way that Ford owns Fiesta cars. The charity is assumed to have a similar expert authority, enhanced by unimpeachable motives, and can therefore present its product to the market in any way it sees fit.' (S Scott-Parker, 1989, p. 11).

This same study also emphasised that the whole process of advertising a charity can be done without disabled people themselves playing any part – other than providing the image which the charity and the advertising agency decide on (and very often even the actor is a non-disabled person). Disabled people are not clients (the charity is), they are not the audience (non-disabled people are – the givers of funds), and they are not the product (the charity is).

The major disability charities are large and powerful organisations. Their exclusion of disabled people from the process by which charities create cultural representations has had significant consequences for us. As Jane Campbell, from the British Council of Organisations of Disabled People, says,

By creating a passive, tragic, dependant image of us, the charities have been able to build their empires. By setting up individual, medical-condition charities (often in competition with each other) and by using harrowing pictures of us plastered on billboards, they are able to raise the cash to build more segregated schools, homes and workshops which, in turn, maintain our image of dependency on them. Their dependency on us for jobs, and above all power, is ignored in this equation (J Campbell, 1990).

Jane Campbell also argues that 'Charities must recognise that their efforts to market "Brand Awareness" of disabled people has pushed them into promoting the medical condition as the cause of disability' (Campbell, 1990). Charities must recognise, she says, 'that the disabilities issue is, fundamentally, one of rights, not charity. Disabled people are systematically forced out of society. Charities must take their share of the blame for this social segregation in that they project through their very influential poster campaigns negative stereotypes of isolated hopelessness.'

Disabled people object to the way we are portrayed in charity advertisements. We object to words like suffer, condemned, confined, victim, and to negative images portraying disability. It is common for a wheelchair to be used as a symbol of imprisonment. This creates two stereotypes. First it translates the meaning of disability into a mobility impairment and makes it even less likely that non-disabled people will recognise and understand other forms of disability. Second, it creates an image of an intolerable life – of confinement, passivity, frustration, and victimisation (all of which can be 'overcome' by plucky little cripples) – instead of portraying a wheelchair for what it actually is, namely a means of mobility, a means of movement, a potential for freedom rather than imprisonment.

If a disabled person, or a disability organisation, complains to an advertising agency about the language or imagery in an advertisement, they are automatically referred to the charity. Susan Scott-Parker found that

> because charities are seen to have legitimate ownership of the 'cause', and because they are seen to be staffed by committed and hard working individuals, disabled people who express dissatisfaction tend to be quietly dismissed and are often seen in fact as part of the problem. They are described as 'ungrateful', 'militants', 'whingers', or most frequently as simply 'ignorant about advertising', too close to the subject and therefore unable to judge. (Scott-Parker, 1989, p. 12).

Disabled people in Britain have recently organised against Telethon, a London Weekend Television fund-raising event. As a television event, Telethon relies on certain images of disabled people, particularly of disabled children. As Ruth Hill says, 'the more pathetic, the more "crippled" we are, the better television we make' (Hill, 1990). Telethon is the ultimate 'lump in the throat' spectacle; the bigger the lump the bigger the cheque. Such an event is predicated on pity and can only deny us our dignity and undermine our rights.

Opposition to Telethon challenges the role which the non-disabled society ascribes to us. Such a challenge happened outside London Weekend Television's studios during the 1990 Telethon. A busload of do-gooders, waving patronisingly at a crowd of disabled people, fell silent in bewildered astonishment when they realised that these were not grateful recipients of charity but angry people telling them to get lost. For disabled people this was an empowering experience whereas to go as individuals, cap in hand, begging for money from an organisation run by non-disabled people takes power away from us (although it may be the only way to get hold of a piece of equipment or a service which is vital to the quality of our lives).

Putting ourselves in the picture

As I have explored, the general culture misrepresents disabled people in a variety of ways. It uses disability for its own purposes, as I have shown above. The films and plays which I have discussed are not about our experiences and our concerns; rather they are about the way that the non-disabled world reacts to disability, what it means to them. Disability thus becomes a metaphor, a vehicle for exploring what is of concern to non-disabled people.

Apart from this exploitation and misrepresentation, disabled people are otherwise missing from cultural representation. Because disability has such strong meanings for non-disabled people, it is difficult for any play, film, book, television drama – even an advertisement – to include a disabled person as a character who just happens to be disabled. The disability would distract the audience or the reader from the role that the character was supposed to represent because non-disabled people generally hold such strong ideas about disability. Disabled people seldom appear in roles where their disability is a secondary characteristic. Directors are reluctant to use disabled actors in such roles so disabled actors find it very hard to get work. Even where roles require the actor to be disabled, it is rare for a disabled actor to be cast – often because the director feels that no disabled actor is good enough for the part (without the opportunities for experience disabled actors are in a Catch 22 position).

Lauri Klobas identifies a few examples of American television – and there are still fewer British examples – where a character just 'happens to be' disabled, but this development is significantly limited by the powerful meaning which is given to visible disability on the screen (Klobas, 1985).

In the early 1980s, disabled people started to pressurise large corporations to include disabled people in their TV commercials. Initial reactions were not encouraging; United Airlines claimed that 'The use of handicapped people would almost inevitably represent an intrusion which could not be explained' and McDonalds said that 'It's a sad fact of life, but if we put them in our advertising . . . people will accuse us of seeking sympathy' (*Disability Rag*, Jan–Feb 1985, p. 7). Nevertheless, following continued pressure by disability activists, three years after this response McDonalds used a disabled man in one of their TV commercials. Throughout the 1980s there was a smattering of American TV commercials where disabled actors were used in 'just happen to be disabled' roles. If we ignore the advertising context, some of these commercials are a joy to watch because of the positive images which come across, although the advertisers have limited themselves to what may be considered to be more 'acceptable' disabilities.

The representation of disability within the general culture in a positive way – that is, in a way which challenges and undermines the current meaning of disability to non-disabled people – partly depends on these kinds of 'happen to be disabled' roles. Unfortunately the emergence of such a phenomenon in the USA is very slow and in Britain it is practically non-existent.

However, it is the creation of a disability culture which is the more fundamental challenge to the cultural representation of disability. The disability movement in both Britain and America has asserted for some years now that, as Sian Vasey puts it, 'we want something more than integration into mainstream culture' (Vasey, 1989). We do need non-disabled people to examine their own prejudices and fears about disability; and we want the proliferation of 'happen to be disabled' roles in television, films, theatre and literature. But we also need to explore our own identity as disabled people. We need to explore what physical and intellectual limitations mean to us, what illness and death mean to us. And we need to explore the experience of oppression common to people with all sorts of different physical and intellectual disabilities – 'through the arts we can make discoveries about what we have in common and place the emphasis on those things rather than on our differences, thus countering the traditional charitable model of disability that has historically kept us separate from each other' (Vasey, 1989).

Deaf people – because they have a separate language – often have a clearer sense of a separate culture and history than do other groups of disabled people. Molly McIntosh told me that, having lived a life of isolation because of her facial scars, she found becoming deaf as a result of meningitis when she was in her late fifties opened a door into a community and a culture which she never realised existed. 'I spent a couple of years after my illness becoming even more isolated and alone,' she said, 'but then I started going to a centre for Deaf people and I suddenly discovered that there was a whole new language [Sign] and a whole new world – once I learned to sign. Now I not only have many friends but I've discovered that Deaf people have a history – reading Harlan Lane's book on the history of Deaf people was a real revelation. And I found that what I look like wasn't really a problem – my communication with other Deaf people is through our language and that's how I relate to people'.

We need a disability culture to give us the confidence to take pride in our difference, to assert that we have an experience which is valid and important. We must challenge the way that non-disabled people interpret our reality by producing our own cultural representations of disability. We need more novels like *The Body's Memory* by Jean Stewart. This book explores the experience of illness and physical disability and the protagonist's development of an identity as a disabled woman. It celebrates the solidarity to be found in joining together with other disabled people to fight oppression and discrimination (J Stewart, 1989).

We need photographers like Mary Duffy, who insists that while disability is central to her work, it also goes beyond disability issues to speak to non-disabled women and to make an impact on the general culture (M Duffy, 1989). And we need poems like the one below by Mandy Dee, a lesbian feminist who was born with cerebral palsy and developed multiple sclerosis as an adult. She died in 1988. Her poem explores a personal experience of disability, illness and death and, by asserting the validity of such experiences, makes concrete the feminist principle of 'the personal is political'.

Night

All my senses are wrapped
In glass, pinched and dry

I look to my past
When I accepted fiercely
the crackle and flashes of light
then my spastic booted
feet crashed thro' the night-street.
So I created minute
earthly sparks to match heaven's stars
and I loved my small striding;
resounding my presence to others –
the quiet walkers
and bland straight standers.

Mostly now my itching creeping senses
comprehend only what my hands and feet
                       can reach.
I lie as if asleep
day by half existent day
in this room
womb of growing multiple sclerosis
tomb of my old strength
life flickering in the darkness.

And I have found a severe delight
that without life death is
uncreated and undead
Death to be must first defer to life.

If the universe and mine utterly
disintegrate
                       and unbecome
death must disperse into chaos
and the root of all creation cease.

So though restrained within one room
and my flashes of defiance
are now restless sclerotic jabs
and hardly painless;
I proclaim
death interspaced eternally
by life, then life.

Suddenly no more stars tonight
Sickness creeps along my spine
I return to the mundane
abandoning philosophy
for warmth and paracetamol
breath out
breath out
breath out.

(Mandy Dee, 1989.)

Chapter 5:
Segregation, Dependence and Independence

The way we live our lives is fundamentally influenced by other people's reactions to our physical and intellectual differences but also by society's reactions to the needs created by those differences. Such reactions will influence, for example, whether we can live in our own homes, have the same educational rights as non-disabled adults and children, what kind of work we do, whether we have access to the same leisure activities as the non-disabled population, whether we can have sexual relationships, friendships, have children, and so on.

The common devaluation of our lives undermines our rights as citizens and as human beings to all the things which are an essential part of a reasonable quality of life. Chapter 2 argued that this devaluation is at the root of the prejudice that we experience and Chapter 4 showed how non-disabled people are generally unable to comprehend our reality in our terms rather than theirs. This disablism, this prejudice, compounded of fear and ignorance, is an important determinant of our social, economic and personal experiences. Disablism takes power away from us; in its extreme form it kills us and, if we live, it can have a devastating effect on the quality of our lives.

Disablism is the ideological part of our oppression. It is integrally linked to the material aspects of the disadvantages we experience. Segregation, the separation from mainstream society, is an important part of the material experience of powerlessness. Segregation takes many forms but comes about because the needs created by our disabilities are not met within society's mainstream activities.

Those who make and implement public policy, whether they be politicians, administrators or professionals, have historically worked within a set of assumptions about disabled people which makes segregation inevitable. For example, the education of physically or learning disabled children has not in the past been seen as part of the role of the ordinary primary and secondary schools; thus physical access and educational support are not on a par with the provision of books, pencils and all the other resources which are recognised as necessary to running a school. This historical legacy means that – even though there is now some recognition of the educational rights of disabled children – parents and children have to campaign for resources which should be available as part of their right to an education.

Segregation also occurs because of the powerless position of disabled people within the market place. The needs generated by our disabilities (physical access, equipment and/or personal support) together with the prejudice generally held about disabled people mean that, unless there is a significant shortage of labour, most employers will be reluctant to take us on. In Britain, only 33 per cent of disabled men and 29 per cent of disabled women under pension age are employed (*OPCS*, 1989, p 69). Disability thus means a likelihood of segregation from the labour market with all the economic powerlessness which that entails.

Finally, segregation occurs because of the association of disability with old age. Retirement from work often brings poverty, and disability is expensive in terms of both housing and personal assistance needs. The difficulty of meeting these requirements brings a high risk of institutional care, heightened by the assumption held by many health and social services professionals that entering residential care is inevitable when someone is both old and disabled.

This chapter looks at the experiences of people who need physical help (by which I mean changes to the physical environment, equipment and/or personal assistance) and the terms on which that help is (or is not) provided. Such people are particularly vulnerable to disablist attitudes – for such attitudes are likely to dictate the nature of the services on which the quality of their lives, and sometimes life itself, depends.

Institutionalisation

In the past the most common form of care provision made for disabled people has been institutions. Institutionalisation is an experience of powerlessness which can grossly multiply the effects of our physical limitations. The disability movement throughout the industrialised world has seen the struggle against residential care as one of the most important parts of the fight for human rights. The Union of the Physically Impaired against Segregation, for example, stated that

> The reality of our position as an oppressed group can be seen most clearly in segregated residential institutions, the ultimate human scrap-heaps of this society. Thousands of people . . . are sentenced to these prisons for life – which may these days be a long one. For the vast majority there is still no alternative, no appeal, no remission of sentence for good behaviour, no escape except the escape from life itself. (UPIAS, 1981, p. 2.)

In their analysis of the literature on all kinds of institutions, Kathleen Jones and A J Fowles concluded that in spite of the disparate approaches of the major writers in this area, there were five findings common to life experienced in a wide range of institutions. They were: loss of liberty; social stigma; loss of autonomy; depersonalisation; and low material standards (K Jones and A J Fowles, 1984, p. 202).

Disabled people argue that these features are as much part of modern day institutions as they were of those in the nineteenth century although the degree to which they are experienced may vary.

I want to look at some of the most devastating emotional and physical abuse which is still to be found in institutions today. Such abuse is an important feature of institutional 'care' for disabled people in many different countries.

In 1989 John Merritt described the situation in which hundreds of mentally ill, learning disabled and physically disabled men, women and children are kept on the Greek island of Leros.

> The smell hits like the reek of an abattoir and the scenes flicker past like some depraved peep show . . . Everywhere are prison bars. In an upstairs cell, bodies lie on beds, naked or wrapped in grey sacking material. Some are curled together, finding comfort in mutual foetal positions, not people but one being. How old are they? 26? 80? A blanket pulled back shows knotted legs. How long has he been there? '24 years.' In the bed? 'Yes, since four years old.' Others are tied, hand and foot to their beds, Why? 'To stop them from falling. (J Merritt, 1989).

In the children's unit, 85 per cent don't leave their beds, because of their physical disabilities. 'Some are strapped down because "they bite . . . " One doctor who visited the children's unit recently said: "Young children with severe handicaps gaze at the ceiling, huddled together, watched by a guard. There is no communication . . . A blind baby was picked up for my inspection. He was five years old. He was put back on the bed to lie, motionless, thumb in mouth, a tiny scrap of humanity totally shut out of human contact." '

Earlier in 1989, Dr Frank Peters and Gerard Vincken, a Dutch psychiatrist and a psychiatric nurse, spent three months on Leros, working with 20 people, beginning to bring them back to life as an example of what could be achieved. They said of the people incarcerated there, 'They were dumped in this isolated place to rot. You might just have killed them then. But most awful is the fact that they are simply waiting until death comes. This is the destruction of the spirit, of the man not the body.' Vincken and Peters quoted Primo Levi who wrote of the Nazi concentration camps, 'Our language lacks words to express this offence, the demolition of a man . . . It is not possible to sink lower than this . . . Nothing belongs to us any more; they have taken away our clothes, our shoes, even our hair; if we speak, they will not listen to us, and if they listen, they will not understand.'

Although conditions in residential establishments in

Britain are no longer physically as bad as those on Leros, many people would argue that their function is the same, namely to look after people who are designated as merely waiting for death, and for whom death would be preferable to life. Disabled people argue that this is the way many of us are treated and that it is a crime against humanity. In contrast, many professionals behave as if people in institutions are socially dead by virtue of the severity of their disability, rather than because of the way society *reacts* to disability. Such an attitude is held by people such as the authors of *A Life Apart*, a major study of British institutions for physically disabled people, which I will discuss later in this chapter.

Many people who were born disabled or who became disabled in childhood experienced significant emotional and physical abuse in institutions during their childhood and carry the effects of this into their adult lives. Ruth Moore described to me her experience of institutions in England in the 1940s and 1950s.

I was four when I got measles and from that I got Still's Disease, which is a form of juvenile rheumatoid arthritis. I was very ill. Between the age of four and 11 I was only out of hospital for about nine months. I was in a general hospital, a children's hospital and a long-term children's hospital. This was by the sea. The treatment was very harsh. A lot of children had TB. Everybody was treated as if they had TB and as if they had to keep the germs away. We had to go outdoors at six in the morning. I think I began to realise then how I was an object. I felt that for years. We were put out in the morning. We were only allowed to wear these pants which had a fastening at the side, and nothing else. Our bedclothes were tightly tucked in at the bottom of the bed and you weren't allowed to put them over you. I had two friends there. We spent most of our days making paper darts and trying to throw messages to each other because half the day you weren't allowed to speak.

I was in quite a lot of pain but it paled into insignificance in comparison with trying to keep in order. It was very

very strict. Like when I had a plaster cast on and I had to stay lying on my bed, you weren't allowed to lift your head off the pillow. And if you did, you had sticking plaster stuck all over your hair and tied underneath. There were all sorts of awful things that only in the last few years have I been able to bear to think about. It was not a good idea to be sick – because you had to eat the sick.

I suppose one of the worst experiences of my life was when the staff took a dislike to this beautiful looking little girl. She had blonde hair. The nurses used to play a game which they used to get groups of us to watch where they held a child under the water in the bath until she started to go blue. And they killed this child. They held her under for too long. I didn't dare do or say anything.

There were three of us who were friends. One of them was sectioned and sent to a psychiatric hospital when she was 16. She was so starved of love. Her mother had had another baby and never came to see her.

I never dared to tell my parents what was going on. All our letters were censored and at the visits which we were allowed the staff were always around – because there were very few visits it was very easy to monitor. My father gave me a doll for my eleventh birthday – I wanted this because I had never had my own toys. I wasn't allowed to keep it.

I was there for 18 months. The other friend who I made there was there for nine years. She eventually worked for the County Council and had access to records about the children who went to the hospital. She did an analysis of all the children who were there while she was and found that two-thirds of them died.

Looking back on her childhood, Ruth wonders how many disabled children were allowed or 'helped' to die, or were murdered, because their lives were deemed not worth living.

How many disabled children have died from neglect and cruelty, with no-one to bear witness to the crime of their life and death? Annie McDonald is someone who, because of the humanity, vision and commitment of a teacher who came across her, was able to write about what was done to her using an alphabet board to point to letters. She was admitted to St Nicholas', a long-stay children's hospital for 'the retarded' in Melbourne, Australia when she was three years old, in 1964. All her limbs are affected by cerebral palsy (they spasm constantly). She also has what is called 'tongue thrust' which means that her tongue goes in and out all the time, making eating and speaking very difficult indeed.

Rosemary Crossley, a teacher who eventually helped Annie to get out of the institution, described her first encounter with Annie, who was then 13 but physically the size of a four year old and who, because she couldn't speak, was assumed to have the mind of a one-year-old child.

> She was lying on her side. The nature of her problem meant that she could not lie on her back [neither could she sit up properly because of her spasms]. Her legs were bent backward, her head and neck were extended backward and her arms were pushed out behind her. She was shaped like a bow, with her arms as the bowstring almost touching her heels . . . Her tongue was going in and out non-stop and she was incredibly, unbelievably thin (R Crossley and A MacDonald, 1982, pp. 20–21.)

Nothing about the way the institution was run was dictated by the interests of the children and young adults (up to the age of 19). Their meal-times were at 7.45 am, 11.30 am and 3.30 pm and they were all put to bed by 5 pm. There was no stimulation, no toys, no activities. Even the television sets were only there for the benefit of the staff.

The cruelty which the children experienced is illustrated by the way they were fed. All of them, even those who could sit up were laid down to be fed.

> Their heads would rest in the nurse's lap, and their bodies would lie across another chair placed in front of her knees. This meant children were being fed with their heads tilted right back, a method called, for obvious reasons, 'bird feeding'; gravity drops the food straight to the back of the throat, and there is no chance to chew. Children were encouraged not to shut their mouths – a second mouthful immediately followed the first. I have filmed a nurse feed-

ing a child: food is piling high on his face because he is unable to swallow it at the rate the nurse spoons it in. It must have been terrifying (p. 11).

In the 1970s, each nurse had to feed 10 children in one hour and, as Rosemary Crossley said, 'everything had to be sacrificed to speed.' By 1980, some improvements in staffing ratios had occurred so each nurse only had to feed five or six children, but the method remained the same. The institution continued to impose emotional and physical abuse on the children even after their practices were exposed in the newspapers and the High Court. They also continued to insist that all the children were 'profoundly retarded', as if this in some way justified their treatment.

Annie wrote of entering a world where there was no affection, no toys, bare white walls, no comfort at all.

The worst thing about going into an institution was the total separation from everything I had known. St Nicolas would not allow parents to leave toys or clothes when they left a child . . . We upset all their rather puritanical ideas about how children should behave. We were not good patients. We cried because we felt abandoned. The nurses didn't know what to do; they didn't know we could feel anguish. The institution had no tally book for broken hearts.

Nurses were discouraged from cuddling children. A crying child needed to be punished for its own good, so it would learn to accept the absence of affection and be happy. Punishment consisted of locking the crying child in a small dark store room. The hospital defined a happy child as a quiet child. Silence was not only golden but sullen; the nurses never saw the looks we gave them when a child was put away (p. 16).

Children like Annie were familiar with death and were aware that their hold on life was tenuous. 'Dying was dependent on the way you felt,' she wrote. The physical care provided was minimal, so 'if you wanted to die you had every opportunity. Many short-stay kids took their chance. Death never appealed to me; I wanted revenge . . . Time was when the strongest emotion I felt was hate, and hate makes you strong. Tender emotions were dangerously softening. Implacable hatred of the whole world which hunted handicapped children into middens like St Nicholas twisted my relationships with people for years' (p. 19).

When Annie was first taken out of the hospital by Rosemary in 1975 she heard people say things like 'Well, if it was a puppy you'd knock it on the head, wouldn't you?' and 'If it was my child I'd kill it and you couldn't blame me' (pp. 82–3). When people looked at her, her twisted and spasming body frightened them. They couldn't conceive of a life being worth living if you looked like that. All her life people had also assumed that she was 'profoundly retarded', and this too was a reaction to how she looked and to the fact that she couldn't speak – at least not a language that they could understand. Rosemary Crossley had assumed that Annie had a mental age four or five at the most and was committed to trying to improve the quality of her life and that of the other children. She had started the kind of play activity with Annie and some other children which non-disabled children of that age would experience and had also started showing them letters and numbers.

But within two months of establishing a way for Annie to communicate, using a board with letters and numbers, Rosemary found out that Annie not only knew how to read and spell but that her knowledge of mathematics outstripped her own. Annie wrote later of the way she had amused herself with numbers during the interminable days before Rosemary found her.

Being physically handicapped alters your expectations of time. You experience total inactivity for such long periods that you become skillful at filling them. During gaps in my life I vied with myself to try my brain against itself, calculating things which I knew existed but whose values I did not know. Being able to see the occasional television programme gave me some ideas. The Bronowski *Ascent of Man* programmes were critical in bringing me in contact with scientific method. In St Nicholas there was not much call for it, but it stopped me becoming intellectually barren. From them I was prepared to use mathematics (pp. 106–7).

Joey was another child at St Nicholas with Annie, who had cerebral palsy and whose speech no-one but the other children took the trouble to understand. Many of the children communicated with each other for years and the staff, including Rosemary, assumed they were making incoherent, meaningless noises. Annie wrote,

When Joey taught us about fractions, suddenly everything started to come together. I started doing arithmetic for fun. I also tried to work out some constants. I had a go at the speed of light, using the distance of the moon from earth (which had been given coverage during the Apollo missions) and the stated delay time for radio signals. My calculation was unavoidably rough, because the time was to the nearest second. I made a stab at calculating the miles per second. I could not convert, because I had no idea how many feet there were in a mile.

Giving pi a value was impossible because I knew nothing about measurement. I could see that there was a relationship between the radius and the outside of circles. I did not know what it was called until later. Getting peak triangles (that is what I used to call two joined right-angle triangles) was easy in a hospital where everyone is in nappies. Bronowski covered Pythagoras, and I had ample opportunity to think about the implications. The hospital nappies were not square and every time the nurses folded a nappy they had to square it first. I became aware of symmetry and its importance in geometry. To calculate I used a crude abacus based on the clock. I used to work in base twelve. I stored the units, treating them as minutes; the twelves I stored on the hour numbers and the grosses I stored on my cot bars.

A knowledge of mathematics rated high in my experience, as it enabled me to occupy myself happily for the later part of my time at St Nicholas. The best bit of work I did was in extrapolating multiplication and division from the addition and subtraction on *Sesame Street*. Multiplication seemed obvious: you added two sets of cot bars together and that meant two thirteens were twenty-six and likewise thirty-twos. Division was harder. I ruined a large part of a stupendous work on A-bombs because I could not divide properly' (pp. 107–108).

The point of highlighting the incongruity between what people assumed about Annie and what was actually going on in her mind, is not to say that she shouldn't have been treated in the way she was because she was not learning disabled. No child should suffer the way the children at St Nicholas' did, and still do at many institutions throughout the world. Regardless of their intellectual abilities, such emotional and physical abuse is outrageous and unforgiveable. All the children in the hospital experienced disabilism in its most extreme form. The underlying assumption was that their lives were not worth living because of their physical appearance and the way their bodies behaved. The staff and the bureaucracy's reaction to their physical and learning disabilities was to set them apart – in both an emotional and a physical sense – from the rest of the world. There was an inability, or a refusal, to empathise with their experience and therefore staff were not motivated to treat them as human beings who could suffer from what was being done to them.

Fear of institutionalisation

Powerlessness characterises the experience of residential care and the nature of institutionalisation affects even those of us who are not in residential care. The possibility of institutionalisation hangs over many disabled people living in our own homes, fuelled by the fear that one day the support which makes our independence possible will disappear, or that an increase in functional limitations will prove too much for whatever resources are available to us.

For Ruth Moore, whose physical abilities are threatened by a worsening of her condition, this fear is very real.

It's beginning to weigh heavily on my mind – the prospect of things suddenly falling apart for me – what would be my option?

Two years ago I broke my leg and the doctor offered to take me into hospital, but I wanted to stay at home. It was towards the end of the seven weeks that I was in bed at home that I started to realise the dangers of my situation. One of the district nurses one night when I had called her out said, 'If you call us out one more time you'll have to go into residential care. If every person that we went to called us back it would be impossible to do our jobs.' I had called her out because I needed the loo and at that point I needed help.

It's an enormous mental strain organising things before you come to them but on the other hand I don't want to be caught in that situation again. There is no way that I will ever go back into residential care. It doesn't matter how nice it seems, you know that your dignity and your identity are going to be stripped from you. It's just such a big issue for me.

Ruth has found that her social worker is sympathetic to her wish to remain living independently. This is an indication of the influence that the Independent Living Movement and the Disability Movement have had on social services professionals over the last 20 years or so. However, most of the people who have campaigned to get out of, and stay out of, residential care have been in their twenties, thirties and forties. There has been little attention paid to those who grow old with a disability. The assumption is often that, once the problems of old age are added to those of disability (particularly because functional limitations may well increase with age), then residential care is inevitable.

Rachel Cartwright's experience bears this out. She has been blind all her life and is now in her 70s.

My husband died last year and since then I've realised how much I relied on him. He used to do all the shopping – not that I couldn't but it was easier for him to go to Sainsbury's and get it all done quickly and bring it back by car. I can't go to Sainsbury's because I can't see all the things out on the shelves. So I go to the local shops where all I've got to do is ask at the counter for what I want. This means I have to do more real cooking! They don't have so many ready-made things in the local shops. I also realised that I relied on him for other kinds of shopping, like if I need a new mop for the floor, or a new kettle, or crockery. With things like that I would have to go to a bigger shop, further away and that means public transport and going into a place which I don't know.

I did feel overwhelmed by things like this, about how difficult it was. And also totally overwhelmed by the paperwork which Jack used to do and which now I've got to get someone else to do for me. Then I had a fall three months ago and broke my wrist. I was admitted to hospital for one night and the following morning they sent the hospital social worker to see me and from the way she was talking, she seemed to think I wouldn't be able to live in my own home much longer. I was so horrified. She seemed to think that it was inevitable I would have to go into a home. But surely it isn't, is it?

Although Rachel's children and grandchildren live nearby they are all at a stage in their lives when putting time into helping her out would pose difficulties. If one of her daughters could afford to give up work then it would be possible for her to help her mother, as well as look after her own children. But Rachel knows how hard up they all are and doesn't want to impose on their lives in this way. She thinks that her children probably don't realise how worried and overwhelmed she feels and that they would be horrified if they knew. 'But why should I put all that on them? It would change my relationship with them all, make me into a dependent rather than the mother and grandmother that I am. I've asked for a home help from the local council but they means test it and I don't think I'm going to qualify because I've got Jack's pension.'

The personal politics of research on institutional care

Most of the general population has very little direct knowledge or experience of residential care. Academics and health and social services professionals play an important role in translating our experiences into beliefs about what residential care means and what kind of services we require. Such people are not immune from prejudice and fear about disability, any more than they are immune from racism or sexism. Just as racism and sexism have been important determinants of how academics and the professions have carried out research and organised services, so disabilism has been a dominant feature of work done by researchers in the fields of learning and physical disability. This is as true for the liberal humanist tradition as it was for the more traditional medical model. As long as an unequal power relationship exists between disabled people and the non-disabled academics and professionals who make a living out of our needs, and as long as prejudice against disabled people is an integral part of our general culture, disabilism will continue to characterise the nature of the research done and the services provided.

Miller and Gwynne's *A Life Apart*, a study of 22 residential establishments for physically disabled people in Britain, is an example of the way prejudice and fear inform research. Published in 1972 but reprinted many times since then, it is a standard text for social work courses; indeed when (as a researcher myself) I sat in on interviews for staff at a residential establishment in 1990 a number of the candidates regurgitated the views put forward in *A Life Apart*.

Miller and Gwynne were obviously somewhat overwhelmed by their close contact with very disabled people during the course of their research, particularly the way that the emotional abuse which disabled people experience often means that we are not the sweet, compliant little souls that the rest of the world would like us to be. They displayed the classic pattern of prejudice against disabled people when they talked about the oscillations of feeling they underwent, being overwhelmed one day by pity for the 'plight of the disabled' and the next day seeing 'the staff as victims of the insistent, selfish demands of cripples who ill-deserved the money and care that were being so generously lavished upon them' (Miller and Gwynne, 1972, p. 7). They experienced great stress 'moving among the disabled inmates and trying to see the world through their eyes' and indulged in the standard defence mechanism of doubting the experiences which were recounted to them, focusing on the individual's psychological state. 'We were subjected to many harrowing stories – of medical mismanagement, of broken promises and rejection, of social deprivation, of physical pain. The historical truth of these stories was unascertainable and sometimes suspect; the acute depression that underlay them was unmistakably true and communicated itself readily to the listener' (p. 7). The authors were so distressed by the imposition of these realities on them that they underwent psychoanalysis during the course of the research (poor things).

Miller and Gwynne had started out believing in the liberal values of what they term the 'horticultural model' of residential care, in which the primary task of the institution is seen to be to develop the potential of each resident, in contrast to the 'warehousing model' in which the task is merely to provide physical care. However, they came to believe that the 'horticultural model' was not appropriate for everybody because some people, particularly those with progressive conditions, find the pressure to maintain or increase independence oppressive. 'Acceptance of dependency may fit the needs of some much better than the struggle against it' (p. 88). More fundamentally, they questioned the validity of both models, arguing that they are essentially 'social defence mechanisms set up to cope with the intolerable anxieties that are associated with the task that society implicitly defines for these institutions' (p. 88). They felt the explicit tasks set (of physical care or encouraging independence) were not real tasks; the real task was 'to help the inmates make their transition from social death to physical death' (p. 89).

Miller and Gwynne argued that if someone had to enter an institution because of physical disability, this meant that 'they are displaying that they have failed to occupy or retain any role which, according to the norms of society, confers social status on the individual.' They claimed this was demonstrated by the way that those who entered such institutions very rarely left. In comparison, criminals and, nowadays, even people who entered psychiatric hospitals were expected to leave sooner or later and to take up some kind of role within society. 'By contrast the boundary of the kind of institution we are discussing is, by and large, a point of no return. It is exceptional indeed for an inmate to be restored to some semblance of a normal role in the wider society. Usually he will remain in the institution, or in another of the same category until he dies' (p. 80).

They went on to highlight the significance of this. 'To lack any actual or potential role that confers a positive social status in the wider society is tantamount to being socially dead. To be admitted to one of these institutions is to enter a kind of limbo in which one has been written off as a member of society but is not yet physically dead. In these terms the task society assigns – behaviourally though never verbally – to these institutions is to cater for the socially dead during the interval between social death and physical death' (p. 80).

Many disabled people would agree that to enter residential care is to be treated as socially dead, to be shut away until physical death. However, we struggle against this, insisting that social death comes about because of the non-disabled world's reaction to disability rather than being an inevitable consequence of even a high level of functional limitation. Miller and Gwynne, on the other hand, believe that for many disabled people social death is inevitable. 'Pressed to its logical conclusion,' they write, 'the real task would imply that the inmate on entering such an institution could be given a capsule that would bring about instantaneous and painless death whenever he chose to take it' (p. 89). Yet again, we are being invited by non-disabled people to 'choose' death rather than the awfulness of living with a physical disability.

Paul Hunt, who was in one of the institutions that Miller and Gwynne studied, was outraged by their belief that disability inevitably meant a lack of social and economic roles and permanent internment in a residential institution (P Hunt 1981). He was also outraged by Miller and Gwynne's assumption that emotional problems were an inevitable part of physical disability. Their research analysed the way in which rejection by society, relatives and friends can have a significant psychological effect on people. However, their message was that this rejection is inevitable and that 'infirmity has psychological – even psychopathological – consequences which are often insidious and even irreversible' (p. 72).

The rejection which disabled people experience is a form of emotional abuse. It has particular consequences for those who are born disabled, or who become disabled in childhood, and who thus experience this abuse from an early age. People who experience such abuse often have what are called 'behavioural problems', just as non-disabled children who have experienced physical or sexual abuse often do. There can be no justification for further abusing such people by shutting them up in institutions and treating them as 'socially dead' (while wishing you could bring about their physical death because they are really so much trouble, and after all their lives aren't really worth living, are they?)

Very few disabled people have had the opportunity to publish their views on residential institutions. We all have strong views on them. 'Whatever background people come from, everyone I've spoken to says they want to move out of residential care,' says Ruth Moore, who has visited many disabled people in institutions. But the views which become part of the general culture are those of academics and professionals working in our field.

An exception to this is Susan Hannaford's study of three residential establishments in Britain (Hannaford, 1985). These establishments were examples of three different types of institution; namely those in which the emphasis is on social and personal development (mainly run by charities but a few in local authority ownership); those in which the emphasis is on nursing care (mainly Young Disabled Units run by health authorities); and those in which the resident is assumed to be in control of his or her life.

There were two features common to all three institutions which Hannaford studied, although their form and impact on the residents differed. First, all the staff at these institutions used progressive words to describe what were in fact oppressive practices. Secondly, the physical environment was in each case a disabling environment (although the degree varied) in the sense that residents were made more dependent than they need have been by the fact that the physical environment had not been appropriately adapted, or the equipment provided, to meet their needs.

Staff at Strode Park, the first institution studied by Hannaford, stated, 'The residents are encouraged to lead full social and personal lives.' In fact the residents' lives served the uses of the charity which ran it, the staff and the surrounding community rather than themselves. Strode Park had previously been called 'Cripple Craft'. It only accepted disabled people who were able to work, turning out goods such as knitted dishcloths and baskets, and being paid nominal wages for long hours. Although the policy was changed in that work was no longer obligatory, residents were seen as 'difficult' if they did not attend the workroom each day and in any case it was a way of passing the time. Some residents were very skilled and the surrounding community benefited from their skills, such as that of a man who repaired antique furniture which was brought in from outside and for which he could only charge a minimal amount.

Residents were made dependent on staff help by the building, which was an old one with few suitable adaptations, by the lack of appropriate equipment, and by the way that the external environment was not suited to their needs. At the same time, help with personal care tasks was given on the staff's terms, organised for the convenience of staff rather than residents. Residents thus had little or no control over when they got up in the morning or went to bed at night, over when and what they ate, over contact with the outside world. Staff seemed to spend more time washing corridors with disinfectant than helping residents with whatever activities they might have wanted to engage in.

Staff thought they were exhibiting kindness and concern by referring to the institution as 'my home' and the residents as 'my boys and girls'. As Hannaford points out, this paternalistic kindness was an inevitable part of the lack of rights and control over their own lives experienced by the residents. The term 'paternalistic' is not used lightly in this sense; the staff took the position of the authoritarian father, who had the right to define the interests of his children and to meet them in the way he saw fit.

When residents asserted their own needs, the reaction was that of a parent to a rebellious child – 'What *is* the matter with you?' – that is, the assumption that the problem lay within the child/resident. The most common form that this took was to assume that the difficult behaviour resulted from someone's failure to 'accept' their disability.

Hannaford also studied a Young Disabled Unit, Victoria House in Margate, which had 20 very disabled people below the age of 65. Although this was a modern building and more physically accessible than Strode Park, the layout of the institution – and the way it was run – had a disabling effect on the residents' lives. There was, for instance, little or no privacy. Most residents had to share rooms and there was only one communal room which served as both dining and recreation room. The toilets for residents' use didn't have doors and instead had curtains which came down to knee level

The institution was run on medical lines, although, as one of the senior staff remarked, 'the majority of residents need no medical treatment'. Nevertheless, the residents' physical restrictions were seen as medical problems. The physical lack of privacy was mirrored in the way that staff freely discussed residents. Hannaford wrote, 'I was treated to a detailed report on these residents' personal lives with a character rundown and their faults discussed . . . Staff seemed to feel that they had a personal understanding of the resident's lifestyle and had the right to comment and make judgements upon it.'

'Troublesome' behaviour, which mainly took the forms of wanting to choose when to get up and go to bed, when to go out, and a wish to leave the institution, was commonly seen in pathological terms. Such behaviour was either explained in terms of a consequence of disability, for example a 'multiple sclerosis euphoria' or in terms of a failure to accept the disability.

The residents' experience of Victoria House seemed to be one of resentment and anger against the constraints and lack of privacy. Such feelings were exacerbated by the feeling that there was no alternative provision for their personal care needs – they were there because no-one could make it possible for them to live in their own homes in the community, and there was no preferable residential option. Hannaford concluded, 'The medicalisation of residents – from their being described as patients, to the medicalisation of disability and the hospital-like regime they are forced to live under – is the cause of many problematic interactions between staff and residents . . .' (p. 59). Indeed, no-one seemed very happy either living or working in such an establishment.

The third institution Hannaford studied, 48 Boundary Road, in the London Borough of Camden, illustrates how the unequal power relationship between disabled people and those responsible for service provision results in oppression even when changes in ideas and provision are motivated by a more sympathetic and humanitarian attitude towards disabled people. We gain something from these advances but the fact that they are made, and their nature determined, by non-disabled people means that they are still part of our experience of powerlessness.

Boundary Road is one of two residential establishments in Britain which are run on the principle of facilitation, which means that the care assistants are supposedly there as the disabled person's 'arms and legs'. The idea is that the disabled person has complete control over their life, what they do each day and how they use care assistants. Founded in the late 1970s, both establishments were run in their formative years by the same (non-disabled) man who had a deep commitment to basic human rights for disabled people.

However, when Susan Hannaford carried out research on Boundary Road two years after it opened she identified a fundamental problem with its seemingly progressive approach. She wrote,

Boundary Road conforms to a social work model. For all its merits, there are drawbacks to this model. Disability tends to be seen within social work analysis; it becomes a social problem. Unlike the charity or medical perspective, disability becomes a social problem surrounding the individual. The individual, then, is exhorted to take control over her/his life with little attention to the structural factors which surround it. The able-bodied position is very different from the disabled one, given existing conditions within society, and to extrapolate from one position to the other is misleading and ultimately puts strain on the disabled individual. Explanations for failure to take control over one's life can all too easily be put down to individual failure. It can become: if you don't succeed at Boundary Road with all the opportunities given you, then you are a failure, a social problem because of your disability and in need of the expertise of a social work staff trained in the inadequacies of individual clients. This is a similar approach to that of poverty, where it is seen in terms of individual inadequacy rather than caused by social factors (pp. 61–62).

Hannaford's research is useful to disabled people, not just for its exposure of the generally oppressive nature of institutions, but also for the way she raises questions about the concepts of dependence and independence. These terms are often applied to disabled people in ways which are against our interests.

Dependence and independence

The issues of dependence and independence are complex but important ones for disabled people. Both terms need thinking about. The word dependence has both negative and positive connotations in that the state of dependence can be associated with helplessness and subordination *or* with reliability. In terms of the physical world, none of us – whether disabled or not – is completely independent in the sense that we rely on nothing and nobody. However, the meaning of our dependence on others and on the physical world is determined by both its socio-economic and its ideological context. For example, we all depend on water coming out of the tap when we turn it on, while a disabled person such as Anna Mathison depends on someone to help her get dressed in the morning. However, when non-disabled people talk about water coming out of the tap, the issue is whether the water company is reliable; when they talk about Anna being dependent on an assistant, the issue for them is what they see as her helplessness created by her physical limitations.

If water does not come out of the tap, the problem is identified as a failure on the part of the water company. However, the nature of the problem when Anna's personal assistant fails to help her get dressed when and how she wishes is determined by the structure within which the service is provided. If Anna pays her own assistant and that assistant fails to do her job properly, Anna may sack her and get another (if she is both confident enough to do this and certain that she can recruit another assistant). If, however, Anna is in an institution then she is unlikely to have the power to decide when and how she wishes to get dressed. Neither is she likely to have that power if the assistant is provided by her local authority and is answerable to a Home Care Organiser rather than Anna herself. When Anna does not have control over the provision of her personal care, the problem is considered to be her own dependence and her demands which do not fit in with the service provided.

If Anna employs her own assistant, the issue for her is whether the assistant is reliable; in contrast, if Anna has little or no control over the personal assistance she needs, the issue becomes her dependence, her helplessness and subordination. This indeed was the case when Anna's helpers were provided by her local council. 'They choose who I have and the times when I can have help. When I need them is dictated for me by the fact that I've got a full-time job and I need to get to work every morning. But the service works to different priorities and they can't or won't be flexible.'

Feminists use the concept of dependency to analyse women's position. In the context of industrialised societies and the family structure found within them, women are economically dependent on men. This economic reliance on men translates into a negative experience of dependency because of the helplessness and subordination that often goes with it. Feminists argue that this dependency is neither inevitable nor desirable and seek ways in which the structures which create women's dependency can be undermined and changed.

In contrast, most non-disabled people, including most feminists, assume that dependency (in the sense of helplessness and subordination) is an inevitable characteristic of a disabled person's life, and stems solely from the fact of physical limitations. A disabled person's reliance on a barrier-free environment, appropriate technology and personal assistance is translated into a helplessness and subordination. What is more, this helplessness and subordination is treated as the issue, as the problem, rather than the issue of the reliability of the environment, of the technology, of the assistance. Thus feminists such as Gillian Dalley (whose work is discussed in the following chapter) use the term 'dependent people' and refer to individual disabled people as 'heavily dependent' with no acknowledgement of the disabilist assumptions which the terms signify.

The word 'independent' also needs looking at carefully. The non-disabled world uses the term in a specific ideological context; it means both physical and emotional autonomy, and the focus is on the individual's ability to achieve this autonomy. When individuals cannot carry out the tasks of daily living for themselves, this is associated with dependence (in the sense of being helpless and subordinate) and independence (in the sense of autonomy) is assumed to be impossible.

Simon Brisenden, who wrote a *Charter for Personal Care* argues that many disabled people are 'victims of this ideology of independence. It teaches us that unless we can do everything for ourselves we cannot take our place in society. We must be able to cook, wash, dress ourselves, make the bed, write, speak, and so forth, before we can become proper people, before we are "independent".' (Brisenden, 1989, p. 9). Those who are born with, or acquire, the type of disability which makes such daily living activities difficult or impossible without help are measured against these standards of independence and if we are found wanting we are consigned to dependence – either within residential care or within our families.

As I discuss in chapter 7, the last 20 years have seen a

steadily growing Independent Living Movement, made up of disabled people throughout the world who seek to establish control over their lives. They also seek to redefine the word independent in a way which will further the interests of disabled people. As Brisenden writes,

> we use the word in a practical and commonsense way to mean simply being able to achieve our goals. The point is that independent people have control over their lives, not that they perform every task themselves. Independence is not linked to the physical or intellectual capacity to care for oneself without assistance; independence is created by having assistance when and how one requires it, by being able to choose when and how care takes place' (p. 8).

Just as it is possible to create the technology and the infra-structure which means that we can depend on the water industry to produce water out of a tap, rather than be dependent on our own efforts for gathering water from a river, so the technology and services can be developed which can change the nature of disabled people's dependency. However, the socio-economic context of our dependency means that our functional limitations are generally treated as the major, and inevitable, constraint and any technology or services developed to address these limitations are delivered with certain conditions.

In capitalist societies, people who are unable to engage in paid work are made dependent – on someone else's pay, on state benefits or services, or on charity. The experience of economic dependence has certain social, political and personal implications. It can create an unequal relationship in someone's dealings with those on whom they are dependent. Whether it does depends on the nature of the relationship. For example, if state benefits are seen as a right, as a necessity to ensure a reasonable quality of life, then the relationship between the bureaucracy which administers them and the recipient will be different from the situation where those on state benefits are seen as having slipped into a 'culture of dependency' and where only the wholly inadequate are unable to 'pull themselves up by their own bootstraps'.

Where a disabled person is economically dependent on a partner, relative or friend, the meaning of this dependence (whether it is the wage-earner's reliability or the disabled person's helplessness and subordination which is recognised) will be determined by the extent to which the relationship is characterised by reciprocity. As I discuss in the next chapter, it is seldom recognised that most relationships involving a disabled person receiving economic and/or personal support from a non-disabled person are reciprocal relationships in which the disabled person is giving as well as taking. This lack of recognition stems from the non-disabled world's inability to see anything except our disability which, to them, means helplessness. So a disabled woman who has young children is seen as a dependent rather than as someone on whom others are dependent.

However, reciprocity is threatened by the economic dependence which is a frequent accompaniment of disability. Clare Robson, who has multiple sclerosis, talked to me about the way that reliance on state benefits means that she cannot contribute as much to her household as she would wish. She and her partner, Mo (who has two children) are short of money and Clare feels that her lack of earning power means that she cannot take an equal financial responsibility. 'Seeing Mo worry about our finances does get to me,' she said, 'I share the worry but feel unable to become involved – because I cannot work. She never criticises me for this. It can't be helped and I know that she hates the fact that I feel, stupidly perhaps, such frustration.'

The importance of the socio-economic context of disability is illustrated by contrasting the situation of two people who are both totally paralysed but whose options and lifestyles are very different.

Christopher Docwra Jones was a young lawyer in 1963 when he contracted polio which left him totally paralysed and using a respirator. He asked the hospital doctor, 'So does the State provide for chaps like me?' and got the reply 'Only if you stay in hospital'. 'Bugger that,' he said and set about using the telephone to do property deals in order to earn himself 'a hell of a lot of money.' (*Observer Magazine*, 21 October 1990). He now owns several homes and has enough money to buy all the technology he needs to create independence for himself. This isn't physical independence for he remains totally paralysed and, for example, can only operate his computer through head movements. But his wealth gives him control over his environment and over how his life and his lifestyle is organised.

In contrast, when Mary Lawson became totally paralysed in 1982 when she was 23, she had no material resources to ensure her independence. Her physical dependence therefore consigned her to a long-stay hospital. The options were very different than those which opened up for Christopher Docwra Jones. 'I didn't think I had a future,' she said, 'I didn't know where I was going to go. My social worker found me a place at the Putney Home for Incurables. She didn't ask me whether I wanted to go, she just said this was the only place for me. She arranged for me to go and visit it, not for me to assess whether I wanted to go there but to see whether they would accept me. It was a huge great place. There were a large number of people there. There were enormous rooms with high ceilings and they seemed bare and clinical. In the far corner there was a television set. I suppose from an outsider's point of view it was clean and well-run but I just couldn't imagine myself living there.'

So, instead Mary went to a hospital run by a religious charitable trust. Here they provided good nursing care but her life was barren and intolerable, She had no control over the daily details of her life, no freedom of movement. She even had no control over the posters on the wall by her bed as the nurses placed religious posters there and Mary did not feel able to ask for them to be taken down. When she eventually refused to attend the religious services which were held on the ward, she was classified as a 'difficult patient'.

Most of us cannot empower ourselves through creating wealth in the way that Docwra Jones did. We therefore seek to empower ourselves through the creation of services which make independence possible. In the past, and too frequently in the present, residential care has been assumed to be the only way that very disabled people can receive practical assistance with daily living. But dependency – in the sense of being subordinate and helpless – is probably an inevitable part of the experience of institutional care, particularly as many people living in residential care feel that they have been declared 'socially dead' (to use Miller and Gwynne's term) and are merely waiting to die.

However, dependence – in the sense of being helpless and subordinate – not only characterises institutional care but can also be part of the experience of living 'in the community'. The most common form of personal assistance is that given by family members. This means that a disabled person becomes dependent on unpaid care and the nature of the care will be determined by the nature of the relationship between the carer and the person cared for.

Anna Mathison spent most of her childhood and adolescence at residential educational establishments for physically disabled people. When she left college, she found living with her mother and relying on her for the assistance she required very difficult. 'It was hard and it was wrong,' she said. 'It was hard in the sense that I was very very independent when I came home. It was hard in the sense that I had lived a lot of my life away from my Mum. I couldn't understand the way Mum was thinking and she couldn't understand the way I was thinking.' Anna had to put up with this situation for some years until, when her mother became sick and couldn't help her, she managed to get a flat of her own from the local council with help from home care workers.

Feminists have identified the family as the location of women's oppression, but it is also too often the location of disabled people's oppression. Such oppression is almost unavoidable in the context of enforced dependence on family members for both material resources and personal assistance. Oppressive relationships can take many different forms. Pam Evans' economic dependence on her father followed the accident which left her paralysed and unable to hold down a full-time job. This dependence meant that his judgements and attitude towards her had greater power to undermine and oppress her.

He imposed on me the obligation to fight my disability, to take on the standards of others which he was totally governed by. He projected his bitter disappointment and resentment of what I had become. For him it was an unmitigated tragedy and he never accepted the new me and was constantly trying to 'improve' me to match the sporty, gung-ho Stoke Mandeville ideal, so that I could at least be put on some sort of a pedestal of achievement. Basically he was trying to compensate for what were his losses, not mine.

When Pam's father died, her mother took over his role in her life.

Taking her cue from my father's manner of monitoring and directing my life, she now became my oppressor also. Being financially dependent on your parents at an age when you've never had the opportunity to establish a life apart from them, tends to ensure that your relationship remains locked in a time warp. You remain a perpetual 'teenager' in their eyes. No concession is made to the fact that you are an adult and in the normal course of events would have left home.

The situation that Pam Evans describes is also a common one for people who are born disabled and have difficulty leaving home, both because of the lack of necessary material resources (housing and access to personal assistance) but also often because of the oppressive nature of their relationship with their parents. Young disabled people commonly find that the only way to escape an intolerable family situation is to enter residential care, or – as Pam found – to marry. In many cases, and particularly in the situation of entering residential care, disabled people are only exchanging one oppressive situation for another.

Disabled people in Britain, in the rest of Europe and the USA, have been campaigning for some years for proper provision of personal assistance services (and this is discussed in chapter 7). However, such services are not generally available in a way that gives us autonomy and maximises our control over our lives. It is the lack of these services which creates our dependence.

In order to promote our interests as disabled people we

have to address the politics of the personal. We not only have to confront the fear and ignorance about the differences associated with disability but also the failure of the non-disabled world to understand – or wish to understand – personal experience of dependency. We want non-disabled people to identify with the experience of relying on others for intimate personal tasks. We don't want them to run away from such a reality because it is too frightening to contemplate.

Feminist theory and research over the last 20 years has given voice to the politics of the personal. 'Community care' for disabled and older people has been a political issue for about the same period of time. The next chapter looks at the contribution feminist thought has made to this area and the implications of this for disabled people.

Chapter 6:
Feminist Research and 'Community Care'

This chapter examines an area of feminist research of particular relevance to disabled people. It is inevitably more 'academic' in tone, though I have tried not to make it excessively so.

Although feminism has generally ignored the experience of disabled women, feminists have actually had a lot to say about the development of social policy on 'community care' – an area of social policy which has a profound effect on disabled people's lives. The feminist concern with 'community care' policies is integrally linked to feminism's central concern with women's position within the family. Disabled people probably shouldn't be surprised – but it is difficult not to feel outraged – that feminist analyses and strategies are entirely from the point of view of non-disabled women.

Feminist theory on the family

During the 1970s and 1980s, feminist academics developed theoretical analyses of the family and of the welfare state. The inter-relationship between the two was particularly apparent in the boom in research and theorising on the issue of 'carers'. Feminists exposed the way that the state exploits women's unpaid labour within the home and the extent to which the policies of caring for elderly and disabled people within the community depend upon women's role within the family.

A key concern for feminists was to assess what social policies should be supported and campaigned for. Research and analysis was particularly directed at the question of whether, and under what conditions, 'care in the community' could be supported or whether alternative types of policy would further women's interests. A theoretical basis for the debate (from a socialist feminist point of view) was set by Mary McIntosh in a contribution entitled *The Welfare State and the Needs of the Dependent Family* (M McIntosh, 1979).

Capitalism, according to McIntosh, depends on a family household system in which 'a number of people are expected to be dependent on the wages of a few adult members, primarily of the husband and father who is a "breadwinner", and in which they are all dependent for cleaning, food preparation and so forth on unpaid work chiefly done by the wife and mother' (p. 155). This system also enables women – whose main role is unpaid caring work within the family, supported by the male wage – to be used as a reserve army of labour when required by socio-economic and technological developments.

The key issue for non-disabled feminists is that this family household system is based on women's economic dependence on men. Mary McIntosh, Elizabeth Wilson and other feminists also identified that the state has an important role to play in perpetuating and strengthening this family system and women's dependency within it (E Wilson, 1977). It followed from this recognition of the role of the state that, if a feminist strategy was to be aimed at freeing women from their economic dependence, campaigns around equal pay and equal employment opportunities were not enough; it was also crucial to resist state policies which perpetuated women's role of providing unpaid labour within the home.

As McIntosh concluded, there were two aspects to the strategy which needed to be developed to address women's role within the family. 'What is called for,' she said, 'is political struggle for state recognition of the needs of both sexes and all unwaged individuals, combined with a transformation of the dependent household so that women can participate in production on the same basis as men.' (McIntosh, 1979, pp. 170–71).

In respect of women's needs as 'unwaged individuals', the work of Hilary Land and others drew attention to the way in which the social security system perpetuated women's economic dependence on men. Various campaigns were waged around specific issues in an attempt to win financial support for women in their own right rather than as wives. This strategy was articulated by the adoption by the British Women's Liberation Movement in 1974 of the 'fifth demand' – that of legal and financial independence.

Feminists also attacked the family as the context in which women provide unpaid care. In the late 1960s and early 1970s the caring function which feminists primarily focused on was childcare. From the late 1970s, however, feminists started to turn their attention to the caring tasks which are carried out within the family other than child care – the care of physically disabled people, of older people and of learning disabled people. This was partly prompted by the fact that during the early 1980s a radical Conservative government enthusiastically took up the issue of 'community care' in its task of bringing about a radical restructuring of the relationship between the state, the individual and the family.

Feminists and 'Community Care'

Caring for people who needed some level of support in their daily lives outside of large-scale institutions had been slowly developing as a social policy since the 1950s, when such ideas had started to be applied to people who were in psychiatric hospitals and asylums. Initially, however, the concept of community was more along the lines of smaller residential establishments within communities to replace the large, isolated asylums which were a legacy from the nineteenth century. Furthermore, for mentally ill people the 'care' that made living outside institutional care possible was primarily the development of certain drugs and also a changing attitude as to what type of treatment was required. It was only when, in the 1970s and 1980s, the 'care in the community' philosophy started to be applied to those who needed physical help with daily tasks, and there was a recognition that most of such care could (and did) take place within families, that researchers and policy makers started to address the issue of who performed these caring tasks.

A piece of research on the care of 'mentally handicapped

people' published by Michael Bayley in 1973, had significantly advanced the debate, identifying the necessity to distinguish between 'care in' and 'care by' the community
(M Bayley, 1973). Bayley asserted that if community care
policies were to be effective, different kinds of professional
services would have to support the care provided by families.
Most people who required physical care had in fact always
had that care provided by families, but the late 1970s and
1980s saw a development of policies which were aimed at
getting those who were in institutional care out into the
community and preventing those within the community from
having to go into institutional care. The provision of domiciliary (home) services, respite care and day care (to supplement
family care) was recognised as a necessary part of community
care.

Policy debates during the 1960s and 1970s had been primarily informed by ideas on institutions and the damage that
institutional life did to individuals – ideas which emanated
from a variety of sources, from the theoretical work of Erving
Goffman to the empirical work of Peter Townsend. However, the development of community care policies in the
1980s have been more determined by the Conservative
government's desire to diminish individuals' 'dependence' on
the welfare state and to emphasise the family's responsibilities for caring. In such a context, feminists and socialists
have been concerned to develop analyses and strategies
which are not merely defensive of the welfare state but which
also promote the interests of women and the working class.

In the context of all this, the feminist research on carers
has been very productive in that it has drawn attention to
the work that women do within the home. This was very
little recognised by policy makers and yet is vital to the
development of community care policies – and particularly
crucial to the Conservative desire to encourage 'family care'
rather than 'state care'.

Mary McIntosh's 1981 article in *Critical Social Policy* sets
out the general terms of the debate which feminists
developed during the 1980s (McIntosh, 1981). Although, in
the context of the Tory ideological and financial onslaught
on state benefits and services, much feminist energy has of

necessity had to go into defending the welfare state, McIntosh argues the importance for feminists of getting our strategic priorities clarified. 'The problem,' she says, 'is whether to press for equality with men, usually in terms of legal, political and citizenship rights, or to press for greater support and respect for women in their role as housewives and mothers.' In other words, 'Should we become more fully proletarianised or should we seek better conditions of dependence on husbands or on state benefits?' (p. 37). McIntosh is arguing from a marxist perspective, but the same question (albeit posed in different terminology) is integral to any type of feminist analysis because of the importance that feminism gives to the role of the family in creating and maintaining women's dependence on men.

Like many feminists, therefore, McIntosh comes down firmly in support of the first strategy – that of placing women on the same footing as men – because this would undermine the dependency relationships within the family. As she writes, 'Women's liberation depends upon the radical transformation of [the] family' (p. 38). The main tactic which McIntosh focuses on in this article is the demand for disaggregation in the social security and taxation system (i.e. the abolition of the treatment of the married couple as one unit for taxation and social security purposes), the motivation being that 'all women will have rights to full social security and that all men will lose the right to state back-up for keeping their wives in dependence' (p. 39). It is no coincidence, however, that in a bracketed aside McIntosh states, 'we should be mounting a much stronger criticism of present ideas of "community care" and fighting for new forms of institutional care that avoid the problems earlier radicals have pointed to' (p. 35). If women's dependence on men and their concomitant lack of economic independence as individuals is grounded in their caring role within the family, then it is but a short step to arguing that women should not do this caring and that such caring tasks should be performed outside the family.

The logic of a feminist strategy on community care policies seems inevitable. As Janet Finch says in an article published in 1984, 'We are clear what we want to reject: we reject so-called community care policies which depend on the substantial and consistent input of women's unpaid labour in the home, whilst at the same time effectively excluding them from the labour market and reinforcing their economic and personal dependence upon men.' (J Finch, 1984.) Finch takes issue with socialists such as Alan Walker (A Walker, 1982) who holds the view that non-sexist modes of community care could possibly be developed through both the expansion of domiciliary services and a challenge to men's attitudes to caring. She argues that even if state provision expanded so that adequate care was provided by paid carers, the family will still remain the setting for community care, and since the family is the location of women's oppression, women's dependence would remain unchallenged.

This leads Finch to ask the question, 'Can we envisage *any* version of community care which is not sexist?' (p. 7). Feminists researching on carers have generally agreed with her when she asserts that she cannot. The case is a strong one; all the evidence is that caring for adults within the home places a greater burden on women and that this caring role is a crucial part of women's dependence. Moreover, as Hilary Graham discusses, the association of 'caring for' with 'caring about' plays an important part in the social construction of what it is to be a woman in Western society (H Graham, 1983). In the context of this analysis, feminists have difficulty supporting community care policies. This creates a dilemma. Either feminists have to support residential care or, as Finch says, conclude that alternative ways of 'looking after highly dependent people' cannot be developed without fundamental social, economic and cultural transformation (Finch, 1984, p. 16).

Finch admits that it may be that 'the only intellectually honest position . . . is to admit that non-sexist caring policies are *not* possible without such a transformation and – until it happens – we must abandon the quest for them, fight other battles, and accept that women will carry on caring' (pp. 16–17.) However, she feels that this position lacks appeal and comes down in favour of the residential alternative. She writes,

On balance it seems to me that the residential route is the only one which ultimately will offer us a way out of the impasse of caring: collective solutions would, after all, be very much in the spirit of a socialist policy programme, and a recognition that caring *is* labour, and in a wage-economy should be paid as such, in principle should overcome some of the more offensive features of the various 'community' solutions. An additional bonus would be for the creation of additional 'real' jobs in the welfare sector.

. . . Working through precisely how such care could be provided in a way which does not violate the relational aspects of caring, nor individual autonomy and identity, and would actually be popular with those for whom it was provided, seems a difficult but a possible programme for both feminists and socialists concerned with this area of social policy. There is a particular urgency about this task, given the rising numbers of elderly people in the population between now and the end of the century (p. 16).

Gillian Dalley has taken up this challenge. In *Ideologies of Caring*, published in 1988, she argues strongly against community care policies and in favour of new forms of residential 'collective' care. She starts from the position that community care policies 'appear to be premised precisely on principles to which feminists are opposed – that is, upon the primacy of the family and the home-bound status of women within it. They are exact contradictions of the collectivist solutions to the problems of caring which feminists would propose' (G Dalley, 1988, p. xii). Dalley not only criticises the failure to provide sufficient resources to enable a good quality of life within the community, but also argues that 'care in the community' is actually against the interests of both women and those people who they are supposed to benefit.

She therefore advocates non-family based solutions to disabled and older people's accommodation and personal care requirements, concluding, 'This much is certain then: the familial model of care which currently dominates is based on premises which are unacceptable to feminists and (often) to those who are themselves dependent on care' (p. 137). Dalley's solutions are to pursue 'alternative' forms of non-family care. For adults in need of physical care, the form of care that she has in mind is primarily residential care (whereas, interestingly, she assumes that non-disabled children will remain living with their parents but that 'collective' provision would take the form of after-school play schemes and day nurseries for pre-school children). This new type of residential care would, accordingly to Dalley, be very different from current residential establishments because the underlying philosophy would be that of mutual concern.

In physical terms there may be little difference – numbers of biologically unrelated individuals live together under the same roof, characterised by some need for care and other support. In one, however, there is a lively integrated community of individuals participating freely and fully in the social life of the group and having relationships with others outside the group, where carers and cared for collaborate. In the other, at worst, there is a collection of separate, isolated, often apathetic individuals warehoused together, serviced by a staff which works in poor and exploiting conditions, having little concern for those in its charge' (p. 121).

Disabled and older people experience daily the inadequacies of 'community care' and would agree with everything that feminists such as Finch and Dalley say about the isolation, poverty and sheer hard work which too often characterises both their lives and that of their carers. However, disabled and older people as individuals and through their organisations have almost without exception put their energies into achieving a better quality of life *within* the community (taking this to mean outside residential care) and have thus maintained a (critical) support of community care policies – whilst recognising that the Conservative government may have some questionable motivations for promoting such policies. For those disabled people who have resisted residential care as the solution to their housing and personal care needs and insisted on their rights to live within the community, the approach of feminists such as McIntosh, Finch and Dalley to care in the community policies is very alarming. Are w right to be alarmed or should we be putting our efforts into demanding better forms of residential care, as they suggest?

'Us' and 'Them'

We can go a long way towards answering this question when we recognise that for feminists writing and researching on carers, the category 'women' does not generally include those who need physical assistance. When Janet Finch asked the question, 'Can we envisage any version of community care which is not sexist?' she went on to say, 'If we cannot, then we need to say something about how we imagine such people *can* be cared for in ways which we find acceptable' (p. 7). In order to understand how she, and other feminists, answer this question it is necessary to recognise who Janet Finch means when she says 'we' and whether 'we' are included in the term 'such people'.

The latter term refers to 'people (of whatever age, although this perhaps is an experience most common in old age) whose physical needs require fairly constant attendance or, at least, the constant presence of another person' (p. 7). Throughout Finch's writing and that of other feminists on community care policies it is clear that the term 'we' quite definitely does not include 'such people'. When Finch and others are assessing what policies would be acceptable to 'us' she means what policies would be acceptable to non-disabled feminists.

Much of the research that feminists have engaged in on caring explicitly separates out non-disabled women from disabled women. Gillian Dalley, for example, refers to 'women and dependent people' as if they are two completely separate groups whose interests, what is more, are in conflict (Dalley, 1988). She introduces her book by saying, 'This book is about dependent people and the women who usually care for them' (p. 1). This separation of 'women' from disabled and older people (who are treated as genderless unless their gender, as in Ungerson's research, is of significance to the carer) is evident in most of the feminist research on caring and has major implications for the questions and issues which feminists consider important. Finch and Groves, for example, identified that the equal opportunity issues around community care were those concerning the sexual division of labour between men and women as carers (Finch and Groves, 1983). In none of the pieces of research is there any analysis of equal opportunity issues for disabled and older women.

This separating out of disabled and older women from the category of 'women' comes about because of a failure of the feminist researchers concerned to identify with the subjective experience of 'such people'. The principle of 'the personal is political' is applied to carers but not to the cared for. This general tendency is articulated by Clare Ungerson's account of why the issue of caring is of personal significance to her. She writes ' . . . my interest in carers and the work that they do arises out of my own biography. The fact that my mother was a carer and looked after my grandmother in our home until my grandmother's death when I was 14 combines with the knowledge that, as an only daughter, my future contains the distinct possibility that I will sooner or later become a carer myself' (C Ungerson, 1987, p. 2). Lois Keith, a disabled feminist, commented on Ungerson's inability to see *herself* (and not just her mother) as potentially a person who needs physical care: 'Most of us can imagine being responsible for someone weaker than ourselves, even if we hope this won't happen. It is certainly easier to see ourselves as being needed, than to imagine ourselves as dependent on our partner, parents or children for some of our most basic needs' (L Keith, 1990).

Ungerson's failure to identify with the interests and experiences of those who need care is then carried over into her feminist analysis. Thus she writes, 'The second set of reasons for writing this book is that it accords with and is fed by my own commitment to women-centred issues and to feminism.' She goes on to identify the 'women-centred' issues around community care.

It has almost reached the dimensions of banality to claim that most carers are women. Nevertheless, given the accuracy of that statement, it seems to me necessary to explore the full implications of the fact. If most carers are women, do women carers feel that what they do is particularly compatible with their female identity? Do men carers feel emasculated? How do women carers feel about caring for men? How do men carers feel about caring for women? There is more to a feminist approach to knowledge than the documentation of the role of women in a set of social processes; while this is important, it is also necessary (and even exciting) to use issues of sex and gender to illuminate those very social processes. The topics discussed in this book are always considered from a gendered perspective; in other words, I have tried throughout to think about the issues by asking the question, do sex and gender make a difference? (p. 2).

Like most feminists who have written on this subject, Ungerson fails to incorporate into her analysis the fact that, not only are most carers women (although, as I shall discuss later, not such a large proportion as feminists have assumed), but so are most of 'the cared for'. Her analysis of social processes involved in the issue of caring must remain incomplete while she considers only one part of the caring relationship and, far from being exciting, research such as hers is profoundly depressing from the point of view of disabled and older women who are yet again marginalised – but this time by those who proclaim their commitment to 'women-centred issues'.

Feminist research on carers is a valuable application of the principle 'the personal is political' and we should not underestimate the importance of the higher public profile of the needs of carers which this research has helped to bring about. However, the failure to include the subjective experience of 'the cared for' has meant that the feminist analyses and strategies stemming from the research have a number of limitations. Most importantly it has resulted in a dilemma being posed between 'care in the community' *or* residential care, which is in many ways a false dichotomy. It is also evident that not only are the attempts to encompass the interests of disabled and older people merely token gestures, but that the interests of carers have not been fully addressed either.

Gillian Dalley's 'Collectivism'

Although Mary McIntosh and Janet Finch were fairly explicit in their espousal of residential care and their rejection of community care policies, neither they nor most other feminists have developed this position much further – they have, in fact, tended to accept that women will carry on caring and that the most that feminists can hope for, this side of the revolution, is better domiciliary support services and respite and day care. However, as discussed above, Gillian Dalley presents a more fully developed feminist critique of community care, arguing for the development of social policy based on the principle of collectivism rather than that of familism and possessive individualism which she says motivates current community care policies.

Most disabled people would thoroughly endorse Dalley's promotion of the principles of collectivism and mutual support – individualism and self-help are not principles that do much to ensure a good quality of life for disabled people. We would also welcome her insistence that disabled and older people should 'be in a position to be responsible for his or her life choices' (Dalley, 1988, p. 115). The problem is that she has reached a decision about which policies should be supported and which abandoned without allowing our voices to be heard.

Like most of the feminist research on community care, Dalley has made no attempt to study the subjective experience of those who are cared for. Instead she undermines our support of 'care in the community' by claiming that either we are merely giving voice to familist ideology or that our organisations are unrepresentative. I want to examine exactly how Dalley ignores our views in order to demonstrate some of the consequences of failing to identify with the subjective experience of those who are cared for.

One of Dalley's reasons for arguing against community care policies is that she believes that these policies are not necessarily supported by 'dependent people'. In arguing this, she refers to a report of the Social Services Select Committee of the House of Commons Report on community care and 'adult mentally ill and mentally handicapped people' which stressed that 'there is still a need felt by many who are dependent for asylum in the sense of haven or refuge, away from the stresses and rigours of the world.' Dalley goes on,

> It may be that many of those stresses and rigours are caused by the prejudice and heartlessness of non-disabled people and that such attitudes should be contested; it is hardly just though to expect the objects of that prejudice and heartlessness to fight that battle themselves from such an unequal and exposed position. It is important, therefore, to recognise the needs and wishes of dependent people themselves; practitioners and policy-makers may be overly susceptible to what the Select Committee report calls 'the swing of the pendulum of fashionable trends and theories' (p. 6).

On such a basis, Dalley insists that community care policies are not necessarily what 'dependent people' want.

Unfortunately, the only evidence that she produces to back up this view is from non-disabled people. The only time she cites the opinion of a disabled person, she quotes him out of context to support a position with which he would never have agreed. In advocating group living for disabled people, Dalley quotes Bernard Brett (whom she describes as 'heavily dependent') on the subject of the advantages of having more than one person providing personal care. 'Nothing is quite as corrupting for all concerned as being completely dependent on too few people,' he says. 'This also tends to exhaust the helpers, who feel under too much strain, and can lead to the risk of various kinds of abuse. I can promise you, there are few less pleasant things than to be cared for by somebody who is constantly tired and under too much strain. This makes life tense, unpleasant and unfulfilled' (quoted p. 120).

Far from advocating some kind of residential, group living situation (which is how Dalley uses this quote), Bernard Brett was describing a set-up where he had bought his own house, let rooms in it to non-disabled lodgers and employed a number of different carers. Like many disabled people, Bernard Brett described residential care as 'a form of living death' and like most non-disabled people he aspired to, and achieved, a home of his own (Shearer, 1982, pp. 37–48).

Bernard Brett was not, of course, receiving 'family care'. He was instead able to choose to pay (in cash and in kind) those who provided assistance to him. However, feminists such as Dalley and Finch have dismissed this as an option to support, arguing that even where assistance within the home is provided by a paid carer, that carer is still likely to be a low-paid, low status woman and, although this is also true for care workers employed in residential establishments, residential workers are more likely to be able to campaign for better pay and conditions. They also, as discussed above, see the removal of caring for disabled and older people from a family setting as a crucial part of undermining women's dependency.

Dalley dismisses the demands that have been made by disabled people and their organisations for good-quality services to enable them to live in their own homes. She insists that either such demands are merely expressions of dominant ideology or they are made by organisations which are not representative of what she calls 'dependent people' as a whole.

She argues that 'Propounders of the familist ideal favour it [community care policy] because for them it embodies notions of the family as haven, as repository of warm, caring, human relationships based on mutual responsibility and affection and thus a private protection against a cold, hostile, outside world (p. 25). When disabled and older people express an aversion for residential care, according to Dalley, this must be set in the context of the strength of the ideology of the family. Where institutional or residential care is available, it is regarded as second best precisely because it differs in conception so markedly from the family model of care' (Dalley, 1987, p. 12). We are invited to treat people's preference for living in their own homes as a kind of 'false consciousness' arising from what Dalley identifies as the 'familist' ideology which pervades our culture.

There is no recognition here that disabled people have often been denied the family relationships that she takes for granted. Insult is then added to injury by the assumption that for a disabled person to aspire to warm, caring human relationships within the setting where most non-disabled people look to find such relationships is a form of false consciousness. We are to be denied not only the rights non-disabled people take for granted, but when we demand these rights we are told that we are wrong to do so.

The other way of undermining disabled people's opposition to residential care – an insistence that our organisations are not representative – should be familiar to feminists. Anti-feminists often seek to undermine feminism by claiming that most feminists are white, young and middle-class. Dalley echoes this sort of divisiveness by quoting a critic of the Independent Living Movement:

> The core constituency of the independent living movement is young, male and 'fit' as opposed to 'frail', whereas a major feature of the social reality of disablement is the elderly female, lacking in robustness and living far from the supportive confines of university campuses [where the American ILM originated]. It may well be that the disadvantages and needs of an elderly arthritic in an urban slum have more similarity to the problems of her able-bodied neighbours than to the values of the movement for independent living (G H Williams, quoted by Dalley, 1988, p. 117).

It is certainly true that the ILM both in the USA and internationally is dominated by men. However, to use this fact to undermine the very principles and aspirations of the movement is to deny the basic human rights for which the movement stands. Dalley refers to the 'heterogeneity of dependency' by which she means that personal assistance requirements are found in a number of different situations, depending on age, type of disability, gender, personal circumstances and so on. This does not mean, however, that the aims of the ILM are only relevant to young, middle class, white men. Such men are merely demanding what young, middle class, white non-disabled men take for granted. The economic and social advantages of this latter group normally enable them to achieve such things – and this is why it is common for white, middle class young men to react with such a sense of outrage and injustice when their social and economic privileges are suddenly threatened by disability. Why shouldn't those of us whose class, race, age, gender and disability mean that we are denied such advantages, insist on the same rights?

Given non-disabled feminists' failure to identify with the subjective experience of disabled and older people, perhaps they should be wary of prescribing the kind of care that would be best for such people. Dalley, however, is not inhibited by this. Dismissing the demands of the Independent Living Movement, she advocates new forms of collective provision on the grounds that it is only by removing caring and servicing functions from a family setting that the sexual division of labour (in both the private and public sphere) will be fundamentally undermined. A skeptical disabled feminist may comment that if communal living is such a liberating force for women, then perhaps non-disabled women should try it first before imposing it on disabled and older women whose lack of social, economic and political power makes them all too easy a target for enthusiasms and fashions in social policy.

Dalley illustrates her case by arguing that a group home would make it possible for a 'bed-bound' young mother to develop an 'ungendered' role. Such a woman, says Dalley, will not expect to 'take up a domestic role vis-à-vis housework and child-rearing as she would (because of normative attitudes at large) if she were able-bodied' (p. 122). Others would perform this role for her and the advantage of a 'collective' setting, according to Dalley, is that her role would be performed by men or women, depending on who was employed.

Such a solution to accommodation and personal assistance needs would be firmly rejected by disabled mothers like Sheila Willis. Her clear aim after learning that she had multiple sclerosis was to remain living in her own home continuing her role of a mother caring for her daughter. Sheila rejected the word 'bed bound' – 'What me? *Bound* to a bed?' During the last two or three years of her life, she spent most of the time on her bed, organising and taking responsibility for not only her own household but also setting up a voluntary organisation which would provide physical help to other disabled people. A feminist for 15 years, her role as a mother and her ability to run her own home were intensely important to her; to deny this would be a denial of her fundamental human rights – and those of her daughter.

Gillian Dalley goes further than most feminist researchers in opposing community care policies but both their and her perspective is fundamentally limited by the common failure to consider the subjective experience of those who are cared for to be a necessary part of the research. Almost all the feminist research on carers treats those who are 'cared for' as passive recipients of that care, and in so doing they also fail to address fully the experience of carers. One (partial) exception to this is Jane Lewis and Barbara Meredith's research on daughters caring for mothers (Lewis and Meredith, 1988). Although this research, like the rest, failed to study the experience of those cared for, Lewis and Meredith had a clear concept of the active role which mothers played in the relationship, and the importance of this for determining the nature of the caring role (see their chapter 4). They were thus able to focus more clearly on the needs of carers. By analysing the relationships between mothers and daughters, and the various factors influencing these relationships (for example both parties' contacts with others), they were able to distinguish positive experiences of caring from more negative ones. This enabled them to identify factors which need to be addressed to mitigate the negative experiences of caring (see their chapter 7).

Unfortunately, however, most feminist research has not properly addressed both sides of the caring relationship. As Lois Keith writes,

In wanting to show how difficult and unrecognised the work of the carer is, many have thought it necessary to portray those who may be in need of care as passive, feeble and demanding. And so deep-rooted are our prejudices about both disabled and elderly people, that no-one really seems to have noticed the damage this can do. It merely confirms what most of us believe about disabled people anyway – that they are more or less helpless and need to be looked after by others. In this debate, they are continuously presented as 'the other', the non-person. They are rarely seen as having valuable lives in the way their able-bodied carer or partner does (Keith, 1990).

Different questions, different answers

Feminists cannot claim to have developed a full analysis and adequate strategies on the issue of community care policies until the subjective experiences of disabled and older people are included within the research. Nasa Begum, a disabled feminist, recently carried out a piece of qualitative research into 10 disabled women's experience of receiving personal care. Her findings illustrate some of the ways that this subjective experience can be incorporated into a feminist analysis of 'community care' (N Begum, 1990). Unfortunately, however, this research is very unusual in that, generally, the feminists who have access to the funds to carry out research are neither disabled nor old and have not, so far, been able to identify with the subjective experience of those who are.

Disabled feminists (were they properly represented within the academic and research community) would raise different questions when carrying out research on community care and would not be faced with the stark choice which Janet Finch has posed between community care or residential care.

Instead of focusing on the 'taking charge of' part of Hilary Graham's definition of 'caring about' (Graham, 1983, p. 13), such research would focus more clearly on the reciprocity involved in caring relationships and the threats to that reciprocity. We would do this because it is the loss of reciprocity which brings about inequality within a relationship – and disabled and older people are very vulnerable within the unequal relationships which they commonly experience with the non-disabled world.

Very little attention has been paid to disabled and older people's experience of physical and emotional abuse within caring relationships. Such abuse occurs within both residential and community care and takes place in the context of physical and economic dependence, where the person being cared for experiences a fundamental inequality in their relationship with those providing physical care. This is an issue which affects both disabled men and women but as Nasa Begum points out, 'Women with disabilities are particularly vulnerable when the practices and assumptions which shape current provision fail to recognise that the nature of the personal care relationship is such that it can legitimise and endorse oppression' (Begum, 1990, p. 41). It is particularly unfortunate that feminism's concern with the various forms of abuse experienced by non-disabled women has generally failed to incorporate the experience of disabled women.

We need to ask whether people want to receive physical care from someone they care about and who cares for them. For Clare Robson, the answer is clear: 'I know that I am loved and that I love her. I feel very privileged and secure. I never, ever, anticipated a relationship that was so wonderful and loving. Obviously there are difficulties. There are, in effect, three of us – me, her and the MS – and we have to take account of the uninvited guest, the squatter.'

On the other hand, Simon Brisenden identified that where there are no options other than dependence on a relative or partner, then this can be 'the most exploitative of all forms of so-called care delivered in our society today for it exploits both the carer and the person receiving care. It ruins relationships between people and results in thwarted life opportunities on both sides of the caring equation' (S Brisenden, 1989, pp. 9–10).

Research needs to examine what makes 'caring for' in a 'caring about' relationship possible in a way which meets the interests of both parties. Many disabled people have clearly identified that 'caring for' in a 'caring about' relationship cannot work unless there is real choice based on real alternatives. Such a choice cannot exist where the only alternative to assistance by a partner or relative at home is residential care.

Where the choice is between unsupported (or minimally supported) 'family care' and residential care, the physical and emotional suffering incurred by both parties to a caring relationship is often enormous. This is starkly apparent, for example, in the case of one of the respondents in Patricia

Owen's study where it was only the provision of services within the home which prevented a disabled mother from being restrained against her will within residential care away from her three-year-old daughter (P Owen, 1987, pp. 21–23). Surely feminists should be supporting strategies which would promote adequate support to people who wish to remain outside, or leave, residential care, rather than washing their hands of community care policies because of the way that such policies currently bolster women's dependency within the family.

Feminist research which incorporated the experiences of disabled and older people might also raise the question of the meaning of the word 'home', separating this out, in a conceptual and political sense, from the feminist critique of the family. Disabled feminists should be able to assert their right to live in their own home without being accused of supporting the oppression of women within the family. Indeed, non-disabled feminists in other contexts have insisted on women's rights to a home (for example, Watson, 1986) yet in opposing community care policies and attempting to undermine the family and women's dependence within it, they are in danger of denying one group of women the right to a home.

Feminist research on caring insists that most carers are women. 'In general,' writes Hilary Graham, 'caring relationships are those involving women; it is the presence of a woman – as wife, mother, daughter, neighbour, friend – which marks out a relationship as, potentially at least, a caring one' (Graham, 1983, p. 15). Disabled feminists would point out that we now know that actually there are 2.5 million male carers and 3.5 million female carers, although women are more likely to be full-time carers (H Green, 1988) and that it is of fundamental concern to (particularly heterosexual) disabled women to challenge the assumption that men will not 'care for' in a 'caring about' relationship.

This assumption is often experienced as oppressive by disabled women when confronted by health and social services professionals who undermine the ability of such women to sustain heterosexual relationships. For example, it seems to be common for married women entering Spinal Injury Units, particularly if they are tetraplegic, to encounter a negative attitude towards the chances of their marriages surviving their disability. One woman's husband was told by her consultant that 'seventy-five per cent of marriages go bang and to get rid of our double bed. I am sure this stayed with him and did not give our personal life a chance. He left 15 months after I came home' (Morris, 1989, p. 83).

Hilary Land has raised the issue of men caring in the context of the increasing trends towards early retirement or redundancy amongst men in the 55–64-year-old age group. 'This means,' she writes, 'that one important legitimate reason not to care, namely that priority should be given to their paid work, is being removed very rapidly from growing numbers of middle-aged men' (H Land, 1989, p. 155). If such men are carers they are most likely to be caring for their wives. In 1986, 46 per cent of British women in the 45–64 age group reported long-standing illness and for 28 per cent their illness limited their activities (*General Household Survey*, 1989, p. 147). We need to know more about the experiences of the significant number of women in both this age group and in older age groups who rely on their husbands for care.

However, it is also of significance that roughly the same levels of long-standing illness are found among British men in these age groups, which must mean that there are many households where both partners require some level of care. Indeed, among the elderly population there is evidence that significant numbers of carers are also in need of care. In this situation we need to know what factors enable or prevent women from getting the care they need.

Feminist research has tended to draw very distinct lines between carers and those who are cared for. This means that the extent to which older and disabled women are also carers is obscured. Lois Keith, in criticising the feminist research on carers, is writing from the perspective of having 'made the overnight transition from someone who was essentially a carer – a wife, mother of two young children, part-time teacher – to someone who was, in addition to these roles, sometimes in need of care' (Keith, 1990). Research on women who have experienced spinal cord injury found that 'women are primarily the carers within a family and most of us continue in this role. Yet too often it is assumed that we will be the passive recipients of care' (Morris, 1989, p. 188). Pam Evans, herself disabled and whose husband has ME, has a positive experience of a reciprocal relationship: 'He looks after me, and I look after him, in complete equality and peace – it's what marriage is in its true sense, a harmonious way of living and a bastion against all external conflicts and demands'.

The failure of feminist researchers and academics to identify with the subjective experience of those who receive care has meant that they have studied caring situations where there are seemingly very clear distinctions between the person who cares for and the person who receives care. Their assumptions have led them to seek out carers and the most common source of identifying potential interviewees is organisations (statutory authorities and voluntary organisations) to whom people have identified themselves as carers. However, a situation in which one party to a relationship has a clear identity as a carer while the other is clearly cared for can only represent one type of caring relationship – and may, in fact, not be the most common. If we focused not just on the subjective experience of those identified as carers but also on the other party to the caring relationship we may find that in some situations the roles are blurred, or shifting. We may also want to expand our definition of caring for to encompass not just physical tasks but also the emotional part of caring for relationships. Research carried out by disabled feminists would, therefore, focus not so much on *carers* as on *caring*.

In their insistence that provision and control over personal assistance services are a human right, disabled people and their organisations are actually mounting a fundamental attack on the family – an attack which non-disabled feminists should be supporting rather than undermining. Simon Brisenden's *Charter for Personal Care* rejects the way in which disabled and older people are forced to look for support from their relatives and partners, arguing that we should receive the financial support necessary to enable us to make free choices about the kind of personal assistance we require

(Brisenden, 1989). Such a demand is not unrealistic, as the introduction in Britain in 1988 of the Independent Living Fund which provides a grant (albeit a means-tested one) to cover the cost of personal care, has shown. Non-disabled feminists would serve us better by joining with us in defending the current government limitations on the ILF rather than assuming that the only way to mount an attack on women's caring role within the family is to consign us to residential care.

Disabled people would join with non-disabled feminists in rejecting the way that 'community care' too often means 'family care'. But we would assert our own political demand – a demand for the right to live within the community in a non-disabling environment with the kind of personal assistance that we would choose. In doing this, we are not only pursuing the human rights of disabled and older people but also launching an attack on the form that caring currently takes. Such a strategy should therefore also be clearly supported by all feminists who wish to undermine women's dependency within the family.

Chapter 7:
Fighting Back

Disabled people throughout history have attempted to insist on their right to live and to a decent quality of life. Even those who were institutionalised under the Third Reich and killed under the Nazi Euthanasia Programme resisted. At Absberg, for example, the residents of the Abbey (an institution run by the Catholic Church for disabled people) refused to get on the bus which came to collect them to take them to the gas chambers. They were dragged and carried by force on to the bus and their resistance put to shame the nuns' and local people's helplessness as they stood by (Gallagher, 1990, pp. 138–145).

The assertion of the value of our lives runs through both our individual struggles with the non-disabled world and the collective action which disabled people have increasingly taken over the last 20 years.

Confronting prejudice

Pam Evans describes her recognition of the assumption that her life is not worth living and the way that this assumption underlies both 'kindly' and hostile reactions to disabled people. It takes courage to confront the fact that this devaluation of our lives is the determinant of most non-disabled people's interaction with us. 'To continue to live as best we can, keeping faith with who we know ourselves to be, in the face of what society has decided we are, does take courage. But it's a quiet, unspectacular and, above all, unrecognised courage. Real courage has no witnesses and no rewards.'

Pam is also generous in her understanding of why non-disabled people so devalue us when she says, 'We should keep in mind when we are being treated in this way, that these things generate from the murkier depths of humanity and that they are not perpetuated consciously. We need to make the effort to understand that people are far more disabled by their attitudes than we are by our physical condition once we acknowledge it unreservedly.'

We have to struggle as individuals on a daily basis against other people's assumptions about us which are such an important factor in determining the quality of our lives. Some of us also have to struggle against racism, sexism or heterosexism. The isolation that Anna Mathison felt as a result of her segregation from mainstream society throughout her childhood and adolescence was compounded by the fact that she was the only Black child at her 'special' school and only one of three Black young people at college. 'I was never allowed to forget that I was a Black child,' she said. 'I remember the hatred, the unkindness. It was difficult to call it racism. It just felt like unkindness, other children being preferred over me when, for example, sweets were being given out. Just little things.'

Anna has fought against disablism and racism all her life. She has asserted herself as an independent, autonomous woman, and now has her own flat, the personal assistance that she requires to carry on her life, and is in paid employment which she enjoys. She has the strength to say, 'I feel very positive about myself and if other people don't recognise my worth then that's their problem.' She sees working with other disabled people as a priority in her life.

Many of us find that joining together with other disabled people brings a feeling of strength. However, when we take collective action together, or organise our own cultural events, we have to fight against the negative connotations of just being together in a group of disabled people. Just as to a white, predominantly racist society, a group of Black youths congregated together spells trouble, so to non-disabled people a group of disabled people are a subject of pity, fascinated repulsion and, sometimes, fear. Such an attitude is undermining and can make us feel uncomfortable about being in a group of disabled people. To overcome these feelings, however, is to feel empowered by joining together.

Rachel Cartwright describes her experience of going to a play put on by a group of learning disabled people:

> I haven't really associated with other disabled people throughout my life, but recently I've started to be involved in my local disability association and there's a strong group of learning disabled people involved in it. They put on a play about the difficulties of leaving home when you're considered to be incapable of independence – and it was brilliant. It felt so good to be in an audience of people with whom I had so much in common – in spite of our age differences and the range of disabilities – and to be listening to something which came out of the experience of being discriminated against because you're different. I remember the difficulties I had establishing an independent life for myself because of being blind but at the time I was just an isolated individual. Whereas these young people are together and angry and saying that they won't put up with it.

Over the last to 10 to 15 years, an increasing number of organisations of disabled people have been formed, which have both broken down our isolation from each other and demanded that the needs associated with our physical and intellectual limitations are met in a way which ensures control over, and a better quality to, our lives.

The Independent Living Movement

The Independent Living Movement started in 1969 when a group of physically disabled hospital residents, who were attending courses at the University of California at Berkeley, organised their own class called 'Strategies for Independent Living'. Rachel Hurst, the British delegate to Disabled People's International (an international federation of disability organisations), explained the origins of the movement when she spoke at a conference on Housing and Independent Living in 1990:

> Despite being in some ways institutionalised by the hospi-

tal, studying and living together had allowed them to form a close-knit group in which their political consciousness could grow. They realised that their need for self-determination and independence was shared by the Black and student civil rights movements which were dominating the university scene in California. And they learned from those movements as well as from each other. They learned where their real oppression lay and took strength from each other in understanding how to deal with it (L Laurie, 1991).

These people faced much opposition in their demand for the right to live independently. There were attempts to expel two of the students from the university on the grounds that their academic goals could not be achieved and that they were not living 'suitable lives'. The students managed to prevent this happening. The principles on which their strategy for independent living was based were seen as a threat to the professionals who made their living out of disabled people's segregation. Rachel Hurst identified the three basic principles involved as: 'those who know best the needs of disabled people, and how to meet those needs, are disabled people; the needs of disabled people can best be met by comprehensive programmes which provide a variety of services; disabled people should be fully integrated into their community.'

She went on to explain how by 1972 the first Centre for Independent Living (CIL) had been established which served both disabled students at Berkeley and disabled members of the wider community. The CIL used a number of different sources of funding to enable people to get access to personal support, accessible housing, advice and information on benefits, an accessible environment, peer counselling, transport and wheelchair repairs.

In Britain where there are now seven Centres for Independent Living, the approach is less on the actual provision of services than on ensuring that local and central government provide the housing and personal and other support services necessary for independent living. The British Council of Organisations of Disabled People has an active Independent Living Forum which forms a network of all the CILs and other organisations of disabled people which are developing independent living initiatives. This forum is also part of a European Network on Independent Living which in turn participates in the Independent Living Committee of Disabled People's International. As Rachel Hurst says, these organisations are all 'rooted in the radical move away from the traditional medical and rehabilitation professionals' control over our lives to the self-help, community-based programmes which ensure our empowerment'.

When the non-disabled society has done things for us it has resulted in our segregation into special schools, residential care and our isolation within a physical, social and economic environment which does not address our needs. Disabled people and their organisations are increasingly insisting that we are the experts on disability and that if we had control over the response to our needs we would develop very different policies from the ones which currently dominate our lives.

The international dimension to the disability movement has brought strength to national movements and is a very important part of the increasing collective organising by disabled people.

Disabled People's International

The First Congress of the Disabled People's International (DPI), held in 1981, adopted a manifesto which set out the organisation's philosophical base. 'We maintain that all people are of equal value. This conviction implies that disabled people have the right to participate in every sphere of society . . . We therefore reject all forms of segregation and we refuse to accept lifetime isolation in special institutions' (Driedger, 1989, p. 54).

The manifesto asserted that disabled people have rights as citizens to education, rehabilitation, employment, independent living and income security. And it also stated that disabled people must have the right to influence governments and policy-makers: ' . . . organisations of the disabled must be given decisive influence in regard to all measures taken on their behalf'.

The significance of disabled people coming together to form an international movement cannot be underestimated. Disabled people are imprisoned within institutions, constrained within inaccessible housing and obstacle-ridden physical environments, dependent on unpaid care by family members, discriminated against in the labour market. Such people lack power by virtue of their socio-economic circumstances. The foundation of Disabled People's International was about disabled people taking control over their lives.

Disabled People's International is also crucial in the struggle against organisations *for* disabled people. In most of the industrialised world, the richest and most prominent organisations working on disability are controlled by non-disabled people and their activities do much to confirm the prejudices against which we struggle. DPI itself had grown out of the conflict with Rehabilitation International, an international organisation made up mainly of (non-disabled) rehabilitation professionals. Until 1980 this was the only international organisation concerned with the needs of people with varying disabilities. Very few disabled people ever participated at its congresses until – following protests by the handful of disabled delegates at the 1976 congress – disabled people in Sweden and Canada organised to increase the number of disabled delegates to the 1980 World Congress and Delegate Assembly. The Swedish delegation put a resolution that organisations of disabled people should have at least 50 per cent of the delegates in a national delegation (which would have meant that at least 50 per cent of the delegate assembly would be composed of disabled people).

When the resolution was resoundingly defeated a meeting of the disabled delegates who were attending the congress was held. The 250 disabled people who assembled decided to form a World Congress of Citizens with Disabilities (which subsequently became Disabled People's International). As two of the Canadian delegates recalled, these disabled people – who came from all over the world – 'had a sense of their own destiny. They wanted to proclaim their rights, as citizens, to an equal voice in the decision-making of services, the policies and programs that affected them. They were no longer willing to passively accept the control of rehabilitation professionals over their lives. They demanded dignity, equality and full participation in society. They demanded release from the yoke of paternalism and charity . . . ' (quoted by Dreidger, 1989, p. 35).

The rehabilitation professionals at the congress reacted either with outright hostility to the idea of disabled people forming their own international organisation or with a condescending paternalism. One non-disabled delegate gave voice to this latter reaction when he wrote, 'To me, they are going through a developmental stage which resembles the adolescent or young adult in a family, who often becomes rebellious for a period of time. After this stage, an excellent partnership and relationship with the "family" evolves and life goes on better than ever.' (quoted by Dreidger, 1989, p. 37).

Against such attitudes disabled people had to assert their autonomy and attempt to take power away from the professionals who controlled not only the disability organisations but also the individual lives of disabled people.

DPI delegates from both developing and industrialised countries found that there were common elements to the struggle between organisations of and organisations for disabled people. Joshua Malinga, for example, recounted the story of the foundation of the Zimbabwean Council of Disabled People and how they were met with hostility. 'When news came out in the papers, we were branded with all sorts of names from all corners. We were called "rebels" and "ungratefuls" . . . They refused to see the difference between an organisation of the disabled and one that is for the disabled. They refused to see the difference between a service organisation and a political organisation fighting for the human rights of the disabled' (DPI, 1981, p. 15).

As in many other countries, the Zimbabwean organisation of disabled people allied itself with the liberation movement. 'As soon as our majority government took over we started meeting all members of the parliament and reminding them that the struggle for liberation, which put them into power, was a struggle for social justice and that it is accepted that the justice should permeate to all communities, including the disabled' (DPI, 1981, p. 16). In South Africa, where the government refused to recognise the International Year of Disabled People, the disability rights movement which emerged in the 1980s soon realised that they had to actively oppose apartheid, both because of the natural links between the struggles of Black people and disabled people as oppressed groups and also because of the relationship between the poverty created by apartheid and the incidence of disability among Black people. As a historian of the movement said, 'The particular handicaps the majority of disabled people in South Africa face are inextricably linked with apartheid. Therefore, in challenging and dismantling these handicaps we also need to do the same to apartheid' (quoted by M Pagel, 1988).

'Organisations of' versus 'organisations for'

Throughout the world, non-disabled people have formed organisations which seek to provide services for disabled people. These organisations operate within a framework which assumes that disabled people are not capable of taking control of their own lives and require the services of professionals and voluntary workers, and the aid of charity. As Mike Oliver, an academic who is disabled, writes, these organisations work within 'the medical rather than a social model of disability which locates the problems faced by disabled people within the individual rather than being contingent upon social organisation' (M Oliver, 1990, p. 115). Or, as Susan Hannaford argued, the assumption is that disabled people are the problem, just as the poor are the problem and not the society that caused poverty, and homosexuality the problem and not heterosexual mores (Hannaford, 1985, p. 82).

Organisations of disabled people, on the other hand, reject the charity and the medical models of disability, asserting that the services we require should be provided as a civil right and that it is society which disables us rather than our physical condition. Organisations for disabled people have their social origins in the surplus time and money of the wealthy and the post-war development of the professions. Organisations of disabled people have very different roots.

Martin Pagel, in his booklet on the history of the disability movement, makes links with the labour and trades union movement both internationally and in Britain. Disabled people in Britain first started to organise during the late nineteenth century. One of the first British organisations of disabled people, the National League of the Blind (founded in 1899; the British Association of the Deaf was founded in 1890), was registered as a trade union and affiliated to the Trades Union Congress.

A movement which asserts the rights of oppressed people to organise for themselves to create better social and economic conditions is bound to ally itself with other oppressed groups – whether these be based on class, race or gender – and is therefore likely to be on the left of the political spectrum. This is undoubtedly one of the reasons for the conflict between organisations of and organisations for disabled people. The latter are run by those who are from the advantaged groups in society (in the sense that they are predominantly white, non-disabled and economically advantaged) and are within a conservative charitable tradition. Governments can afford to give financial and political support to such organisations for they do not challenge social, economic or political frameworks.

Those disabled people who ally themselves with organisations *for* disabled people do so predominantly because their class position leads them to fear radical social change. Some of us may feel a sense of outrage at how such disabled people are used to give legitimacy to the organisations which do so much to oppress disabled people. We must also recognise, however, that internalised oppression exerts a tremendous influence. A disabled person who holds a position within a conservative charitable organisation has been told all their lives – as we all have – how inadequate and pitiable disabled people are. Small wonder then that such people, when asked to involve more disabled people in their organisation, commonly respond that there just isn't any capable person with the relevant expertise amongst the disabled community.

Just as some women who achieve high social and economic status take on the role of an honorary man and often do little to further the interests of other women, so some disabled people take on the role of honorary non-disabled people. They are considered to be exceptions to the rule of the inadequacy of disabled people generally. In accepting this role they do little or nothing to aid other disabled people and in giving their support to organisations *for* disabled people they do much to confirm our oppression.

The British Council of Organisations of Disabled People is the British branch of the DPI. It is made up over 80 organisations controlled by disabled people and as such it is engaged in a struggle to wrest control and resources away from the disability charities. In 1990, RADAR, the major umbrella group of the organisations for disabled people, received just under £500,000 from the Department of Health. In comparison BCODP received £30,000 – but then BCODP has an unequivocal commitment to policies such as anti-discrimination legislation which, if implemented, could have major resource implications. Such a policy is also predicated on the notion of disabled people having civil rights rather than being recipients of charity; this too constitutes a fundamental challenge to the prevailing ideology.

Racism, sexism and heterosexism

Disabled people and their organisations are no more exempt from racism, sexism and heterosexism than non-disabled people and their organisations. While DPI has made strenuous, and to some extent successful, efforts to ensure that developing countries are fully represented, within its constituent national organisations both women and ethnic minorities are distinctly under-represented and issues around racism, sexism and sexuality have tended to be avoided.

At a national conférence held in Britain in 1990 on housing and independent living, Millie Hill addressed the issues for Black disabled people. 'Black disabled people, I have found to my cost, are a discrete and insular minority within a minority. We have been unfairly and unjustly saddled with restrictions and limitations, subjected to a history of purposeful unequal treatment and relegated to a position of political powerlessness and disenfranchisement in a society where even the label "second class citizen" seems wholly inadequate to identify our social status' (L Laurie 1991). The discrimination which all disabled people face, she said, is compounded for Black people by the discrimination that Black people face in areas such as employment, housing and education. The disability movement needs to address issues such as the way that services for disabled people are predominantly provided by white non-disabled people for white disabled people.

At the same conference Michael Jeewa from the Asian People with Disabilities Alliance argued that Black disabled people need, at present, to organise separately from white disabled people. This does not mean, however, that the white-dominated disability movement can abdicate its responsibility to address the interests of Black disabled people. Indeed, there are integral links between racism and the discrimination that disabled people face, as was made clear by a remark Sir Geoffrey Howe made when he was Foreign Secretary. He was responding to the demand that people from Hong Kong should be given the right of entry to Britain before the takeover of the former British colony by China in 1997. 'Any society,' he said, 'has a limit to the pace at which it can absorb people, and the more strange they are the more difficult it is to accept them.' Such a remark can be equally applied to non-disabled people's reactions to those whose physical or intellectual differences mark them off from the normal.

The disability movement also has a responsibility to address the interests of disabled women. Non-disabled academics tend to think that they are addressing such interests by highlighting how much worse off disabled women are than disabled men (and how much worse off Black disabled people are than white disabled people). There is something very offensive about this type of analysis because essentially such academics are assuming a right to define our reality – and it is predominantly a very negative reality from their point of view. We, too, must not fall into the same trap of treating issues around women and disability, race and disability, sexuality and disability (or, indeed, class and disability) as things to be 'added on' to our history, our politics and our organising. The experiences of Black and ethnic minority disabled people, disabled women and disabled gay men and lesbians are integral to the experience of being disabled. Disabled people, as a group, are made up of Black people, women, gay men and lesbians as well as of white people, men and heterosexuals. Sexism, racism and hetero-sexism affect us all and the struggle against them must be an integral part of any disability politics.

The meaning of disability

Academics and professionals play a key role in influencing the meanings which non-disabled people give to disability and in determining the policies and services which affect our lives. The models of disability which most commonly inform this role are the 'personal tragedy' and medical models of disability. Those who subscribe, consciously or uncon-sciously, to these models view disabled people as individuals whose experience is determined by their medical or physical condition. Someone who is blind is thus viewed as experienc-ing a 'personal tragedy' and it is the role of the professional to mitigate the difficulties caused by not being able to see. The individualist assumptions which are at the heart of this definition of disability also encourage a particular psychology of disability. By this I mean that disabled people's behaviour is often interpreted in terms of individual pathologies. Our justifiable anger about our oppression is interpreted as a self-destructive bitterness which arises out of a failure to 'accept' our disability. Our difficulties in getting access to the resources we need to live independently are treated as a 'lack of motivation' or similar individual inadequacies.

The medical and 'personal tragedy' models of disability and the attitudes which go with them are a very important part of the powerlessness experienced by disabled people in their relationship with those professions whose role is so important to the quality and nature of our daily lives. Dis-abled people – in their struggles to assert their autonomy and to counter their powerlessness – challenge these attitudes in their day-to-day contact with those who have power over us.

In our attempts to challenge the medical and the 'personal

tragedy' models of disability, however, we have sometimes tended to deny the personal experience of disability. Disability *is* associated with illness, and with old age (two thirds of disabled people are over the age of 60), and with conditions which are inevitably painful. The Liberation Network of People with Disabilities, an organisation which made an explicit attempt to incorporate the politics of the personal, recognised this in their policy statement. This included the point that, unlike other forms of oppression, being disabled is 'often an additional drain on the resources of the individual, i.e. it is not inherently distressing to be black, whilst it may be to suffer from painful arthritis' (*In From the Cold*, June 1981). To experience disability is to experience the frailty of the human body. If we deny this we will find that our personal experience of disability will remain an isolated one; we will experience our differences as something peculiar to us as individuals – and we will commonly feel a sense of personal blame and responsibility.

This sense of blame was something that Clare Robson experienced in respect of other people's attitudes towards her physical condition. She had multiple sclerosis for years before she received medical confirmation of it. During that time, there were all sorts of pressures on her to deny her illness and what was happening to her body. Nobody wants to be ill or to have a body which doesn't work properly. We all find it difficult to confront another's pain and physical difficulties. After she received final confirmation that she had multiple sclerosis, Clare realised that many of her friends had assumed that her physical symptoms had been psychologically motivated. She says, 'One interesting piece of information that came to light after I told people that I had MS was the opinions that they and others had had of me. I guess that I was both hurt and mildly angry to discover that I had been seen as a lazy and work-shy person.' Clare had for some years experienced exhaustion and found it difficult to hold down a full-time job. The realisation that other people had seen her physical difficulties as a personality inadequacy led her to say, 'I was just left feeling betrayed by friends of many years.'

It is, of course, less frightening for others to explain our physical difficulties in terms of personality inadequacies – it is yet another way of saying that it couldn't happen to them.

When illness and physical difficulties – and old age – are so associated with personal inadequacies and are so painful to confront, it is also easy for us, in our attempts to assert control over our lives, to insist that we are young, fit and competent. The truth of the matter is that most disabled people are not young, are not fit, and have great difficulty in developing the competence to control our lives. This last factor is primarily a result of our material experiences and the effect that these have on our confidence and self-esteem, but developing the ability to take control of our lives is not immediately and automatically brought about solely by the provision of favourable material circumstances.

Someone like Mary Lawson, for example, not only has to deal with the lack of material resources, which makes her life very difficult, but also with the effects of years of institutionalisation, which have undermined her personal sense of worth. Mary has taken other people's tendency to blame her for her situation into her own way of seeing things, and feels that it is her own inadequacies which led to the people around her – primarily health and social services professionals – writing off her future.

She said, 'I think the hardest thing to cope with while I was in hospital was the idea that I picked up from the people who worked there that they were sacrificing themselves by helping disabled people; that this was a very unpopular thing to do, and that coming to work with disabled people was a sacrifice.' In summing up her difficulties in living independently Mary said, 'It's a non-story really. It's a waste of time talking about it. I've made terrible mistakes. It's my fault that people around me didn't want to help me – I wasn't able to provoke feelings in other people that would mean they wanted to help me.'

Material resources and personal support can make a major difference to Mary's life. However, we also have to recognise that, however positive she may feel in the future, this will not alter the fact that she is paralysed, and that this paralysis brings various physical complications. We are doing ourselves no favours if we deny the physical difficulties which go with being disabled.

Rachel Cartwright, having carried on most of her life 'as if I weren't blind', now recognises that growing old brings physical changes and restrictions which she can't, and in fact now doesn't want to, deny:

> I realised that when I was younger I was refusing to look after myself in the way that I needed to because I was saying that being blind didn't make any difference to me. I spent a while getting very angry with growing old and hating it. Now I feel more friendly towards my body and feel that I want to look after it by recognising that I'm slowing down, that I can't do so much now as I used to. But I feel good about this because I feel I'm more in touch with the real me.

The experience of ageing, of being ill, of being in pain, of physical and intellectual limitations, are all part of the experience of living. Fear of all of these things, however, means that there is little cultural representation that creates an understanding of their subjective reality. The disability movement needs to take on the feminist principle that the personal is political, and in giving voice to such subjective experiences, assert the value of our lives. We can insist that society disables us by its prejudice and by its failure to meet the needs created by disability, but to deny the personal experience of disability is, in the end, to collude in our oppression.

Positive images

Over the last few years disabled people have tried to counter the negative images that are so commonly used to portray our lives with images that convey a sense of strength and control over our lives. It is very important to challenge the standard representations of disability. For example, most pictures of disabled people – whether used to illustrate articles in social work journals or fundraise for charity – present us as pitiable, un-able, marginalised. Such representations fundamentally undermine us.

However, there are problems with what we mean by a positive image of disability. In asserting that not all disabled women are in their seventies and eighties but that some are younger and may have children, it is easy to suggest that being a young mother (in spite of being disabled) is a form of being normal and socially acceptable whereas being old and disabled is not. However much our lives may approximate to those who are not disabled, we are not normal in that our physical or intellectual abilities mean that we do not conform to the norm, the average.

For myself, I do not want to have to try to emulate what a non-disabled woman looks like in order to assert positive things about myself. I want to be able to celebrate my difference, not hide from it.

Our history is hidden from us, as are role-models to whom we can relate. Because the presentation of our experience is controlled by non-disabled people, most of the recording of the lives of disabled people is done in a way which is deeply alienating to us. When the life of a disabled person is publicised in a supposedly positive way it is generally done in such a way to set them up on a pedestal, setting them apart from the rest of us by the 'isn't she or he wonderful?' attitude. All of us experience difficulties because of our disability and we all struggle against these difficulties. We can draw strength from the experiences of others but only as long as they are not set apart as exceptional.

Ruth Moore, who survived the awful experiences of residential care that she described in chapter 5, has struggled throughout her life against the powerlessness that results from the prejudice and hostility directed against disabled people. Her strength is an inspiration to us – but only if her experiences are presented in her terms and not those of the non-disabled world.

Having spent most of her childhood in long-stay hospitals, Ruth ended her teens with little education and no preparation for adulthood.

By the time I was nineteen, they couldn't do anything else

for me surgically. So I went home. Then it was a question of my father telling me what I should do. He got me into Queen Elizabeth Training College (a residential further education establishment for disabled students) and I lasted ten days. I fell and broke my arm because there was no help around one day when I needed to go to the toilet and I slipped. I lay in bed in the dormitory for a week with my arm broken. That was the start of agoraphobia because I was down in this dormitory all day alone. The sister used to come in the middle of the day to give me a bed pan. I just felt that I was completely alone, the worst isolation I had ever experienced. I couldn't do anything. There was no way of communicating with anyone. On the Monday they decided to send me home in an ambulance.

In those days the cab and the back of ambulance were divided off and the ambulance attendant raped me in the back on the way home. So by the time I got home I was in a terrible state. And I couldn't tell anyone about it. I never told anyone until I started seeing a counsellor recently. My life was worth nothing – that's what it all meant to me.

Many of our experiences – whether they are of physical or emotional abuse or just prejudicial attitudes – tell us that our lives are worthless. Ruth, however, had not written her own life off.

I advertised in the local adult education newsletter and I got someone to come and teach me shorthand and typing over four years. My father said I had to pay for it and he got me a job in his firm adding up invoices. I did this at home, in my head, eight or ten hours a day. It earned me a little money and it paid for my tuition. I always think, when people say to me, 'Oh you're so lucky,' let me tell you that I have worked for everything I've got.

Eventually, after four years when I had passed all the exams, I decided to start my own business teaching other people shorthand and typing. I put my advert in the paper and people came to me. I worked either mornings or afternoons and every evening and Saturdays. I did invoices in between. I did that for seven years.

Of course what I was doing, and I realise now how effectively I did it, was that I shut myself off from having to face the rest of the world. I sat behind a desk so no-one ever had to see even the whole of me. I had agoraphobia for two of those years. I used to think of any ploy not to go out. Occasionally I had to go out but I felt so ill.

Eventually Ruth got over her agoraphobia and got a job working for her local health authority. By then in her thirties, she wanted to live away from her parents but found that the only way she could do this was to go back into residential care. 'I couldn't find anywhere for ages. In the end I went into the Royal Hospital Home in Streatham because it was the only place where I could get a room to myself. I had to pay over all my income and only kept six pounds per week.' But, after all those years of living with her parents, she was at least able to start taking decisions for herself and this eventually enabled her to get a flat of her own with the personal assistance she needed – after putting much pressure on the local authority. Ruth now runs her own consultancy and has travelled all over the world, furthering the cause of disabled people's demands to live independently.

It is through the experience of someone like Ruth Moore that another disabled person can draw strength to fight her or his own battles. We can also draw strength from the fact that many disabled people have thought deeply about the nature of our experiences and of prejudice and have much to offer in making sense of our lives.

Pam Evans, for example, in describing the impact of prejudice, asserts the importance of naming our oppression: 'Many of us will affirm that the constraints and discomforts of our disability are child's play when compared to the imposition of *gross* preconceptions and assumptions made about us without any consideration for our feelings or recourse to our opinions.' We have to develop a language to make sense of this experience. Otherwise, she says, 'we are powerless to explain it to ourselves, let alone fully understand that it is generated from the outside and not from the condition per se.' Naming an experience of oppression is a crucial beginning of the struggle against it.

Once we have found a language to describe our experience, from our point of view rather than that of the non-disabled society, we can assert the experience of disability on our terms. An important part of this is not just identifying the way that society disables us and struggling for our civil rights, but also identifying the positive experience of disability.

A number of the women I interviewed for this book see disability as a positive thing to have happened to them. Pam, who became disabled when she was 18, told me,

> Not all of us view our disability as the unmitigated disaster and diminishment that seems expected of us. We know that what hurt, anger and distress we have felt was not generated by the condition itself but by the obstacles and offensive assumptions that society heaps upon it. If we dare express the view that it has brought spiritual, philosophical and psychological benefits, it is suggested that we are making a virtue of necessity, repressing our pain, or glorifying suffering. Such certitudes generally issue from those whose experience of necessity, pain or suffering is considerably less than our own and who, above all, have no personal experience of our condition.

To Pam, the experience of not being normal has been a liberating one. 'If we can appreciate that to be an outsider is a gift, we will find that we are only disabled in the eyes of other people, and in so far as we choose to emulate and pursue society's standards and seek its approval.' She warns against the strong pressures to adopt the non-disabled world's standards.

> We need to keep a wary eye on our own motives. Proving something to ourselves can be a disguised way of seeking the praise and approval of others; of proving ourselves to be normal. While we share society's view of disability it's the obvious way to proceed: we've all done it. Indeed in the young or newly disabled of any age, it's virtually

unavoidable. It is so horrible to be patronised as an inadequate write-off that it's small wonder if we seek achievement, praise and reassurance of our normalcy. At the time it feels so much better to be regarded as courageous and marvellous than pitiful. But it is a double-edged sword that forces us into the self-publicist, over-achieving, 'see how normal I am' trap, no matter how society may approve of it. Do we really want the doubtful honorific of being an 'inspiration' to others? Stuck up there on the bloody pedestal, is that any more integrated than the rubbish-bin at the other end of the equation? It's certainly not the liberty some of us seem to think it.

Clearly we need to be able to function in a sociable and balanced manner to pursue a career, earn a living or simply get on with whatever circumstance we find ourselves in. What we don't have to share, or tolerate, is the belief, however grudging, that the standards of the able bodied are superior and the only ones available. 'Normal' does not equal 'right, good and positive'. Fighting to fulfil some ideal of normalcy is only another form of compensatory behaviour that gives power to the nonsense that to be average is to be better than that which is not.

Once we can put aside any need to prove ourselves equal to the able-bodied, cease to do battle *against* ourselves, cease to be brave, stoic or resigned, we can then accept ourselves unreservedly as implicitly equal, able to go beyond the limits others impose on us. Once we cease to judge ourselves by society's narrow standards we can cease to judge everything and everyone by those same limitations. When we no longer feel comfortable identifying with the aspirations of the normal majority we can transform the imposed role of outsider into the life-enhancing and liberated state of an independent thinking, constantly doubting Outsider who never needs to fight the physical condition but who embraces it. And by so doing ceases to be disabled by it.

As Micheline Mason wrote in *In from the Cold*, a magazine produced by the Liberation Network of People with Disabilities, 'There is an essential common core to all liberation movements: the right to be both different and equal' (M Mason, 1982, p. 18). We can celebrate, and take pride in, our physical and intellectual differences, asserting the value of our lives. And while confronting the very real difficulties that physical and intellectual differences involve, we can fight against discrimination and insist that the needs created by those differences are met in a way which enhances the quality, and our control, of our lives.

Chapter 8:
Pride

Last night I joined a demonstration against the BBC's 'Children in Need' event which raises money for 'disadvantaged' children every year. It was organised by the Campaign to Stop Patronage, a group of disabled people who oppose the way that the charity system uses negative images of disabled people to raise money for things which we should receive as a right, instead of having to beg, conform with and show gratitude to patronising organisations over which we have no control.

It was a cold, dark, November evening and we gathered on the pavement opposite Television Centre in West London. A steady stream of commuters' cars rushed past us while over on the other side of the street adults and children queued to get into the BBC, eager to demonstrate their kindness and generosity towards those less fortunate than themselves.

Being part of a group of obviously disabled people, shouting our anger across the road at those who think that all they are doing is being kind to us, is a unique experience. Most importantly, it feels very powerful, much more powerful than I ever felt on a trade union, Labour Party or women's movement march back in the days when I could walk. I first felt this sense of power when I joined the anti-Telethon demonstration in the summer of 1990 outside London Weekend Television studios. Then, it seemed so *incongruous* that here were 50 or so people whose physical difference means that the non-disabled world mostly reacts to us with pity and revulsion, taking over the pavement and eventually the road, producing a lot of noise with the aid of a microphone, enjoying ourselves and our solidarity with each other while challenging the role that society has assigned to us.

The incongruity is really driven home when people don't at first realise what we are there for. At the anti-Telethon demonstration, groups of people would arrive fresh from carrying out any manner of silly stunts, clutching their cheques and cash, broad smiles on their faces when they saw what they thought were a group of the poor disabled welcoming them to the television studios. As they got closer and they realised that we were shouting angrily at them, chanting 'Rights not Charity', their faces would drop and a stunned silence would fall over them. None of them ever knew how to respond; it was so unexpected because they had swallowed so completely the line which the charities put out about doing good for those less fortunate than themselves, who would in turn be so grateful.

We caused a lot of disruption and embarrassment at that demonstration. Neither the police nor the television company's security guards knew how to react when confronted by a group of women in wheelchairs blocking the path of a 'celebrity' as she tried to get to her car. 'Are we going to move them or not?' muttered a security guard in desperation, 'I wish someone would take a decision.' For a while they seemed afraid to touch us – in case we had a fit or something equally terrifying, I suppose. By the time of the 'Children in Need' demonstration, the police had learned their lesson and they kept us firmly on the other side of the road, although this did not stop some of our number crossing over and handing out leaflets to the baffled members of the public whose reaction can only be described as an unhappy astonishment – after all they thought they were helping people like us, and here we were being so ungrateful.

The obvious challenge that we were mounting to people's assumptions was also a source of my sense of power. Indeed, each time I had to explain to a non-disabled friend why I was going on such a demonstration, I was very conscious of the way that this issue challenges the root of our oppression and that even to explain my motivations very briefly brings people up short against the core of their own prejudice.

And yet, in the midst of feeling strong and united with other disabled people, secure in the knowledge that the challenge we were mounting was crucial to the fight against our oppression, one person was able, with one gesture, to negate my strength. Two men came up to us, thinking that we were part of the 'Children in Need' event. One of them offered me a £5 note, which I refused, giving him a leaflet and explaining that we wanted rights not charity. He stopped short, realised with a shock what I was saying and then said that he agreed with me and he had never thought about it quite like that before. In the meantime, the other man had also offered a £5 note to someone behind me. She accepted it; she was fed up at that point of explaining the message yet again and we were collecting money for the Campaign anyway. Having given her the money, this second man turned to go. As he passed by me, he stooped down, patted me on the head and cupped my cheek in his hand, smiling benevolently as he did so.

As Nabil Shaban said (in his film *The Fifth Gospel*, made for the BBC's Everyman series), in response to a similar experience, 'The biggest problem that we, the disabled, have is that you, the able-bodied, are only comfortable when you see us as icons of pity.' Our disability frightens people. They don't want to think that this is something which could happen to them. So we become separated from common humanity, treated as fundamentally different and alien. Having put up clear barriers between us and them, non-disabled people further hide their fear and discomfort by turning us into objects of pity, comforting themselves by their own kindness and generosity.

It is this response which lies at the heart of the discrimination we face – in employment, in housing, in access to all the things non-disabled people take for granted.

It is this which lies at the heart of a refusal to accept that the denial of these things is a civil rights issue and not a result of individual inadequacies. And it is this response which motivates the whole charity industry – all those people making money and fame out of us, and individuals like the man who patted my head, making himself feel good by being kind to someone who he thinks is so much worse off than him.

Moreover, it is the assumption underlying this response, that our lives are of such little worth, which we struggle

Griffin, Susan, (1982), *Made from this Earth*, The Women's Press.

Grimshaw, Jean, (1986), *Feminist Philosophers*, Harvester Wheatsheaf.

Hannaford, Susan, (1985), *Living Outside Inside*, Canterbury Press, Berkeley, California.

Hansell, Susan, (1985), The Wolf, in Browne, Connors and Stern (eds), Cleis Press, San Francisco.

Hill, Ruth, (1990), Grant us some Dignity before your Donations, in *The Observer*, 2 September.

Himmelweit, Sue, (1988), More than 'A Woman's Right to Choose'?, in *Feminist Review*, 29, Spring.

Hunt, Paul, (1981), Settling Accounts with the Parasite People: a Critique of *A Life Apart*, in *Disability Challenge*, 1, UPIAS.

Johnson, Mary, (1990), Unanswered Questions, in *Disability Rag*, September/October.

Jones, K and Fowles A J, (1984), *Ideas on institutions – analysing the literature of long-term care and custody*, Routledge Kegan Paul.

Keith, Lois, (1990), Caring Partnership, in *Community Care*, 22 February.

Kent, Deborah, (1988), In Search of a Heroine: Images of Women with Disabilities in Fiction and Drama, in Adrienne Asch and Michelle Fine, *Women with Disabilities: Essays in Psychology, Culture and Politics*, Temple University Press.

Klobas, Lauri, (1985), Here's Looking at You, in *Disability Rag*, Jan–Feb.

—— (1987), Hollywood, in Sam Maddox (ed), *Spinal Network*, Sam Maddox and Spinal Network, Colorado.

ambert, Sandra, (1989), Disability and Violence, in *Sinister Wisdom*, 39.

nd, Hilary, (1989), The Construction of Dependency, in Bulmer, Lewis and Piachaud (eds), *The Goals of Social Policy*, Unwin Hyman.

rie, Linda, (1991), National Conference on Housing and dependent Living, Shelter.

s, Jane and Meredith, Barbara, (1990), *Daughters Who e*, Routledge.

against every day of our lives. While non-disabled people devalue our lives because of our physical or intellectual differences, we have an uphill battle for the resources which are the real determinants of the quality of our lives. The demonstration outside Children in Need was part of that struggle, for we didn't look like people whose lives were worthless. We looked like people who enjoyed each other's company, enjoyed the music and the jokes we created. We looked as if we took pride in ourselves.

On my way home, I stopped my car to let a woman across a zebra crossing. She was a black woman in her sixties or seventies struggling across the road with the aid of a walking stick, her legs and feet swollen and her back bent. This was one of the poorest parts of London, and she looked like one of its poorest inhabitants. She was more representative of the majority of disabled people than I am – or indeed than any of the rest of us on the demonstration. Yet the challenge that we are mounting to the way that disabled people are perceived and to the discrimination we experience speaks as much to her life as it does to mine.

Bibliography

Armstrong, Keith, (1982), Vernichtung Lebenswerten Leben, in *In From the Cold*, Liberation Network of People With Disabilities, Spring.

Bayley, M, (1973), *Mental Handicap and Community Care*, Routledge Kegan Paul.

Begum, Nasa, (1990), *The Burden of Gratitude*, University of Warwick and SCA.

Blackwell-Stratton *et al*, (1988), Smashing Icons: Disabled Women and the Disability and Women's Movement, in Michelle Fine and Adrienne Asch, *Women with Disabilities: Essays in Psychology, Culture and Politics*, Temple.

Bolte, Bill, (1990), Thoughts on the Death of an Actor, in *Disability Rag*, September/October.

Bowles, G and Klein D, (1983), *Theories of Women's Studies*, Routledge.

Brisenden, Simon, (1989), A Charter for Personal Care, in *Progress*, 16, Disablement Income Group.

British Medical Association, (1988), *Euthanasia*, BMA, 1988.

Browne, Susan, Connors, Debra, and Stern, Nanci, (eds), (1985), *With the Power of Each Breath*, Cleis Press, San Francisco.

Bunch, Charlotte, (1988), Making Common Cause: Diversity and Coalitions, in Christian McEwen and Sue O'Sullivan (eds), *Out the Other Side*, Virago.

Campbell, Jane, (1990), *Who is in control?*, paper presented at the Cap-in-Hand Conference, February.

Crossley, Rosemary and MacDonald, Anne, (1982), *Annie's Coming Out*, Penguin.

Dalley, Gillian, (1987), Women's Welfare, in *New Society*, 28 August.

_____ (1988), *Ideologies of Caring – Rethinking Community and Collectivism*, Macmillan.

Davis, Alison, (1989), *From Where I Sit*, Triangle.

Dee, Mandy, (1989), Night, in *Sinister Wisdom*, 39, Winter 1989–90.

Disability Rights Education and Defense Fund, (1982), *No More Stares*, DREDF, Berkeley, California.

Disabled People's International, (1981), *Proceedings of the First World Congress*, DPI.

Driedger, Diane, (1989), *The Last Civil Rights Movement*, Hurst.

Duffy, Mary, (1989), Cutting the Ties that Bind, in *Feminist Arts News*, Vol. 2, No. 10, Spring.

Farrant, Wendy, (1985), Who's for Amniocentesis? The Politics of Prenatal Screening, in H Homans (ed), *The Sexual Politics of Reproduction*, Gower.

Finch, J, (1984), Community Care: Developing Non-Se[xist] Alternatives, in *Critical Social Policy*, 9.

_____ and Groves, D, (1983), *A Labour of Love – Wo[men,] Work and Caring*, Routledge and Kegan Paul.

Finger, Anne, (1991), *Past Due: A Story of Disabilit[y, Preg]nancy and Birth*, The Women's Press.

Franchild, Edwina, (1985), Untangling the Web [...] in Susan Browne, Debra Connors and Nanci S[tern,] *With the Power of Each Breath*.

Fuss, Diana, (1989), *Essentially Speaking – Femi[nism] and Difference*, Routledge.

Gallagher, Hugh, (1990), *By Trust Betrayed: [..., Phys]icians, and the Licence to Kill in the Thi[rd Reich,]* Holt, New York.

_____ (1985) *FDR's Greatest Deception, [...],* York.

General Household Survey, (1989), HM[SO.]

Graham, Hilary, (1983), Caring: a La[bour of Love, in Finch] and Groves.

Green, H, (1988), Informal Car[ers, General Household] Survey 1985, Supplement A, HM[SO.]

Longmore, Paul, (1987), Whose life is this, anyway?, in Sam Maddox (ed), *Spinal Network*, Spinal Network and Sam Maddox, Colorado, USA.

_____ (1990), Interview, *Link*, ITV, September 1990.

Mason, Micheline, (1982a), Life: Whose Right to Choose?, in *Spare Rib*, 115, February.

_____ (1982b), Employment – a right to work? in *In from the Cold*, Liberation Network of People with Disabilities, Spring.

MacDonald, B and Rich, C, (1983), *Look Me In The Eye*, The Women's Press.

McIntosh, Mary, (1979), The Welfare State and the Needs of the Dependent Family, in S Burman (ed), *Fit work for women*, Croom Helm.

_____ (1981), Feminism and Social Policy, in *Critical Social Policy*, 1.

Merritt, John, (1989), Greece's Bedlam, in *The Observer*, 10 September 1989.

Miller, E J and Gwynne, G V, *A Life Apart*, Tavistock.

Morris, Jenny, (1989), *Able Lives – Women's Experience of Paralysis*, The Women's Press.

_____ (1990), *Our Homes, Our Rights*, Shelter.

Morrison, E, (1989), Editorial, in *Feminist Arts News*, Vol. 2, No. 10.

Oliver, Mike, (1990), *The Politics of Disablement*, Macmillan. OPCS.

Owen, Mary Jane, (1987), A Romp through Metaphor Land, in *Disability Rag*, Jan/Feb.

Owen, Patricia, (1987), *Community Care and Severe Physical Disability*, Bedford Square Press/NCVO.

Pagel, Martin, (1988), *On Our Own Behalf – an Introduction to the Self-Organisation of Disabled People*, Greater Manchester Coalition of Disabled People.

Proctor, Robert N, (1988) *Racial Hygiene: Medicine Under the Nazis*, Harvard University Press, Cambridge, Mass.

Ramazanoglu, Caroline, (1989), *Feminism and the Contradictions of Oppression*, Routledge.

Reiser, Richard, (1990), Resource Cards 12 A and B: History – Disabled People in Nazi Germany, in Richard

Reiser and Micheline Mason, *Disability Equality in the Classroom: A Human Rights Issue*, ILEA.

Rome, JoAnne, (1989), Untitled, in *Sinister Wisdom*, 39.

Rose, Hilary, (1987), Victorian Values in the Test Tube: The Politics of Reproductive Science and Technology, in Michelle Stanworth (ed), *Reproductive Technologies – Gender, Motherhood and Medicine*, Polity Press.

Saxton, Marsha, (1984), Born and Unborn – the Implications of Reproductive Technologies for People with Disabilities, in Rita Arditti, Renee Duelli Klein and Shelley Minden, *Test Tube Women: What Future for Motherhood?*, Pandora.

—— and Howe, Florence, (1988), *With Wings*, Virago.

Scott-Parker, Susan, (1989), *They aren't in the brief*, Kings Fund Centre.

Sereny, Gita, (1977 edition), *Into that Darkness: The Mind of a Mass Murderer*, Picador.

Shearer, Ann, (1982), *Living Independently*, CEH and King's Fund.

Sjöö, Monica, (1972), A Woman's Right over her Body, in Michelene Wandor (ed), *The Body Politic*, Stage 1.

Spelman, Elizabeth V, (1990), *Inessential Woman*, The Women's Press.

Stanley, Liz and Wise, Sue, (1983), Back into the Personal or: our Attempt to Construct 'Feminist Research', in G Bowles and D Klein, *Theories of Women's Studies*, Routledge.

Thompson, Dai, (1985), Anger, in Browne, Connors and Stern, *With the Power of Each Breath*.

Stewart, Jean, (1989), *The Body's Memory*, St Martin's Press.

Sutherland, Alan, (1981), *Disabled We Stand*, Souvenir Press.

Ungerson, Clare, (1987), *Policy is Personal*, Tavistock.

Union of Physically Impaired against Segregation, (UPIAS), (1981), Editorial, *Disability Challenge*, 1, May.

Vasey, Sian, (1989), Disability Culture: It's a Way of Life, in *Feminist Arts News*, Vol. 2, No. 10, Spring.

Walker, A (ed), (1982), *Community Care: the Family, the*

State and Social Policy, Oxford, Blackwell/Martin Robertson.

Walker, Ivy, (1988), A Doctor's Story, in *New Society*, 8 April.

Watkins, Bari, (1983), Feminism: A Last Chance for the Humanities? in G Bowles and D Klein, *Theories of Women's Studies*.

Watson, Sophie and Austerberry, Helen, (1986), *Housing and Homelessness: a Feminist Perspective*, Routledge Kegan Paul.

Waxman, Barbara, (1990), Interview, *Link*, ITV, September 1990.

Williamson, Judith, (1990), It's Hell on Wheels, in *The Guardian*, May 10.

Wilson, Elizabeth, (1977), *Women and the Welfare State*, Tavistock.